RENAL DIET COOKBOOK FOR BEGINNERS

300+ Kidney-Friendly Recipes to Recover Your Kidney Failure and Start Living Again, Including a 28-Days Meal Plan to Organize Your Meals and Avoid Dialysis.

Sandy Moon

1

Table of Contents

5

6

7

9

VEGETABLES 296

Introduction

Chronic kidney disease is a term used to describe how a person's kidneys gradually fail, resulting in more and more dialysis treatments. In earlier times, when a person had kidney disease, they would be confined to a hospital bed. With the advent of dialysis machines and kidney transplantation, it is possible to manage kidney disease at home.

Living with renal disease doesn't mean that you have to give up eating food. You can still eat practically, but you'll need to change some of your habits and become more familiar with the renal diet. As with any diet or weight-loss strategies, it's essential to follow a routine to stray from your practice. When it comes to chronic kidney disease, lifestyle changes and renal diet can help you survive kidney failure. The Renal Diet Cookbook for Beginners is full of advice to manage your condition.

Kidney health is a significant part of overall health. Chronic kidney disease is no joke and can be fatal if it is not managed correctly. The Renal Diet Cookbook for Beginners gives you the knowledge needed to start working on your kidney disease. Some bad habits can influence your kidneys, but some good habits can help you lower blood pressure and increase blood flow to your kidneys. Below I have written down some tips that can help you with chronic renal disease and other topics related to kidney health.

The Renal Diet Cookbook for Beginners is designed to give you the tips, ideas, and inspiration you need to manage and treat chronic kidney disease – also known as CKD.

Chronic kidney disease (CKD) is a severe condition that can cause kidney failure. There are two types of CKD: Chronic renal failure, caused by damaged kidneys, and kidney function loss; Congestive heart failure leads to an inability to get enough oxygen into the body, called hypoxia. To control chronic kidney disease symptoms, it is necessary to know which foods are suitable for the kidneys and which kinds of food you should avoid. This book will give you tips about managing CKD, everyday habits that can lead to kidney problems, and more.

This book aims to make you understand how necessary it is to monitor your diet and adjust it to your needs. The renal diet, as we said, is recommended for people suffering from chronic kidney disease and consists, for example, in regulating protein intake. The result will be that you will need fewer dialysis treatments or kidney transplantation.

If you are new to the system of renal diet, I will guide you through the process.

The goal of a renal diet is to prevent protein wasting by reducing the workload of your kidneys. This means that with a renal diet, fewer toxins are being produced in your body. This improves your overall health, increases energy levels, and reduces inflammation. It also helps you recover from illness faster, which will allow you to delay dialysis for more extended periods. You will notice that your overall hunger will reduce while following a renal diet.

You can follow a renal diet to manage your chronic kidney disease without too much difficulty. You should be aware of various things, though: This book shows you how to incorporate a kidney diet into your lifestyle to live a healthier life. It has recipes that are easy to follow with simple instructions. Each recipe will give you a complete breakdown of all the nutrients that it contains so that you can monitor your health while still eating delicious food!

You will also find a 4-week meal plan that will help you stay focused and be less stressed about starting this new journey.

Understanding Chronic Kidney Disease in Our Health

CKD (Chronic kidney disease) is a disease that occurs when the kidneys fail to function correctly and are not able to take off toxins from the blood. It is a common and progressive health condition that affects millions of people in the United States. According to the National Kidney Foundation, approximately 80 million Americans have pre-dialysis CKD, while another 18 million have post-dialysis CKD. For every person with pre-dialysis CKD, there are between 12 and 15 additional people with post-dialysis CKD.

In the United States, CKD affects older adults and minorities at higher rates than Caucasians. Recent research suggests that the racial disparity in CKD is since persons of African ancestry are more likely to suffer from diabetes, an aggravating factor in kidney failure development.

According to the National Kidney Foundation, CKD is a disorder that is silent in its early stages. This means that persons experiencing CKD have no symptoms until they begin losing kidney function. Approximately one in three people who have pre-dialysis CKD will eventually need a kidney transplant before they die. Other individuals will need dialysis or lifelong renal replacement therapy (RRT).

What Are the Symptoms of Ckd?

There are many symptoms of CKD. The main ones to look for are swelling in the hands and feet; increased blood pressure; loss of appetite; weight loss; fatigue; nausea; abdominal cramps and pain; frequent

17

urination; dark urine or uremia, or urine appears brown or orange. However, kidney failure may not cause any symptoms until it is too late to do anything about it. The symptoms of chronic disease may not become apparent until later stages. When CKD begins early in life, there may be no noticeable symptoms at all. However, the damage is already done if you are no longer able to produce enough urine. You may need to undergo dialysis or take medication to ensure that your kidneys usually function again. Many people diagnosed with chronic kidney disease remain unaware of their condition until their health worsens significantly. This is because they do not experience any symptoms, and their kidneys begin to deteriorate slowly over time. Many people who have the renal disease don't even know it yet because they may not experience any symptoms right away. If they experience symptoms, they'll probably think they're suffering from some UTI or digestive problem. While this is true in most cases, it's a good idea to check with your doctor about your symptoms because sometimes kidney damage isn't apparent until later in the disease process.

What Are the Causes of Ckd?

There are many causes for CKD, including diabetes, high blood pressure, high cholesterol, kidney stones, obesity, and heavy smoking.

The effects of chronic kidney disease vary from patient to patient. Some people will experience symptoms while others will not. If you think you may have CKD, talk to your doctor about getting tested to see if you have a problem. Chronic kidney disease (CKD) is a catch-all term for several specific conditions affecting the kidneys. These disorders can cause chronic pain, low blood pressure, and poor kidney function. These symptoms are often mistaken for other diseases and health conditions because they do not follow an obvious pattern or course.

When a human has chronic kidney disease, the kidneys do not function as they should. Some of the most repeated causes of this condition are diabetes, obesity, hypertension, hyperparathyroidism, high calcium levels in the blood (hyperkalemia), and some medications. We should know that a healthy lifestyle can lead to a healthier body. But for some, it doesn't come easily. Chronic diseases like cancer and diabetes can leave a person unable to eat the foods they used to love.

If you feel that your diet lacks some of your favorite foods, you might be in the early stages of chronic kidney disease. Chronic kidney disease is a chronic disease that can lead to a loss of kidney function and even death. If you have a urinary tract infection, which, if left unchecked, will trigger kidney damage, you should seek medical advice right away. It's just as necessary to make adjustments to your lifestyle to take medication. It may help alleviate many of the root causes of kidney failure by following a healthier lifestyle and eating healthy.

You should:

- Lower the consumption of high salt, high potassium, and phosphorous
- Control diabetes through insulin injections
- Should not eat foods high in cholesterol
- Consume heart-healthy diets such as whole grains, fresh fruits, low-fat dairy products, and vegetables
- Increase physical activity at least half an hour a day
- Leave smoking
- Limit your alcohol consumption
- Try to lose excess weight

- Control your fluid intake

Kidney disease ordinarily will not go away once it's diagnosed. The best way to keep your kidneys healthy is to acquire a healthy lifestyle and healthy eating habits. Over time, kidney disease can get worse. It could also contribute to the failure of the kidneys. If it is not treated on time, kidney failure may be life-threatening. When the kidneys are partially functioning or not functioning at all, kidney failure happens. This is monitored by dialysis. Using a pump to remove waste from your blood, your doctor may prescribe a kidney transplant in severe instances.

Hence, to keep your kidneys healthy, you must eat kidney-friendly healthy food less in potassium, phosphorus, and sodium, since kidneys filter out all the toxic waste from food.

Who Runs the Risk of Having a Ckd?

In healthy people, the kidneys can maintain a constant amount of filtrate in the blood, regardless of whether the person is growing or not. However, in people who have chronic kidney disease (CKD), the regulating filtrate is lost. This leads to an enlarge in the amount of blood that contains too much protein and blood glucose. This condition is known as proteinuria and raises the risk that urine will include a higher protein concentration than average.

It can lead to diabetes and heart problems, increasing one's susceptibility to developing other illnesses such as liver disease, lung disease, high blood pressure, and cancer.

Kidney disease can also be acute or chronic. In acute kidney disease (AKD), either the kidneys fail suddenly and entirely, or they fail slowly over a short time. However, there is an ongoing loss of kidney function with chronic kidney disease over years or even decades.

For adults older than 65 years, the incidence of chronic kidney disease rises. There is a greater chance of experiencing kidney failure in persons with diabetes. Diabetes, responsible for approximately 44 percent of new cases, is the primary source of kidney failure. If you have this disease, you will also be more likely to get other diseases.

Some chronic kidney disease risk factors include:
- Diabetes types 1 and type 2
- High cholesterol
- Obesity
- High blood pressure
- Kidney failure
- Kidney cancer
- Cigarette smoking
- Obstructive kidney disease
- Liver failure
- When urine flows back into the kidneys (vesicoureteral reflux)
- A narrow artery that supplies the blood to the kidney
- Bladder cancer
- Heart and blood vessel (cardiovascular) disease
- Vasculitis
- Family history of kidney disease
- Autoimmune disease
- Abnormal kidney structure
- Older age
- History of chronic kidney disease in the family

People with CKD are at risk for:
- Peripheral neuropathy
- Erectile dysfunction
- Alzheimer's disease
- Heart attack
- Stroke
- Glaucoma

The Assistance of Renal Diet

The renal diet is a special type of optimal protein diet used to help prevent kidney disease. For those unfamiliar with chronic kidney disease, the kidneys are responsible for flowing out toxins in the body through urine. They help people maintain a normal amount of fluid in their bodies. However, when they do not function properly, those functions are hampered, and toxins are not removed from the body. This can show serious health issues such as hypertension or high blood pressure, diabetes, heart disease, and even death.

Unless there is an acceptable reason you should eat more protein than your kidneys can safely handle, the renal diet is ideal for you. Why? Because it lets you eat anything you want while avoiding any foods that will put your kidneys at risk. Kidneys have very little ability to break down very many foods, so they will not be able to process them well if they are present in your diet. This can lead to high levels of protein in your urine. In turn, this can lead to several other medical issues if not corrected.

When someone has chronic kidney disease and needs to eat regularly, there are many options, including a renal diet. A renal diet is a simple term of an optimal protein and low-sodium diet prescribed by a medical doctor to help patients with chronic kidney disease avoid the use of dialysis.

If you have recently been diagnosed with Chronic Kidney Disease, you may be unsure about the types of foods that are best to eat. After all, you probably don't feel like eating much these days.

The renal diet is a nutritious diet that helps people who have kidney failure stay healthy while on dialysis. This book will help you answer out what foods you can eat and what foods you can't eat while on dialysis.

What Are the Benefits of Following a Renal Diet?

Following a renal diet will help you to lose weight by controlling renal function, that refers to the vital parts of the kidney. The kidneys are essential organs that play a crucial role in maintaining life and regulating hormones' balance. The renal diet plan is an optimal protein, low-sodium, and low-carbohydrate diet that helps lose weight by restricting carbohydrates, sodium, and calories and adjusting the amount of proteins. There are many benefits to renal dieting, including the following:

the protein intake is reduced, which is a crucial point to consider; dietary protein stimulates enzymes needed for blood filtration and can reduce the effects of kidney disease and its medications; the food choices are restricted; therefore, lowering cholesterol and allowing for less chance of heart problems. It helps reduce blood pressure. It also reduces the chance of complete kidney failure or dialysis machine dependency. It helps prevent cancer because the body contains more oxygen and energy when there is less protein in the body.

The renal diet is a lifestyle that helps people with chronic kidney disease to maintain good health. Some of the amazing benefits of the renal diet are:

- Reduces Risk of Chronic Kidney Disease and Death
- May Improve Liver Health
- Helps Avoid Dialysis Use

- Increases Overall Well-Being
- Improves Quality of Life
- Improves Quality of Life for Children and Parents of Patients with Kidney Failure
- May Prevent Dietary Protein Toxicities in Children with CKD
- May Help Support Ketosis and Ketogenic Diet in Children with CKD
- Provides Safe, Balanced, Nutrient-Dense Food Intake
- Provides a Safe Food Supply for People with CKD
- Provides a Safe and Healthy Diet for People with CKD
- Provides Safe, Nutrient-Dense, and New Foods for Patients on Renal Dietary Programs
- Provides a Safe and Nutrient Dense Diet for People with CKD

How Can the Renal Diet Avoid the Use of Dialysis?

Chronic kidney disease (CKD) is a global problem. Millions of people agonize from this condition every year. Some people are fortunate enough to notice the signs right away, but many others have little to no symptoms. A renal diet is your strategy to avoid dialysis while eating a nutritious diet but low in protein. While on a renal diet, your blood is made a little thinner with each meal because your kidneys aren't working as hard to filter out toxins and extra chemicals from your blood.

This is one of the reasons that dietary protein can be a problem for patients with kidney disease. While on a renal diet, it is common to have a protein deficiency, which means that protein will then be used for other body functions like muscle growth or building new blood vessels. The renal diet is a very healthy and balanced diet, with all the necessary nutrients to maintain good kidney health. The main motive of the renal diet is to avoid the need for dialysis. You can consume any food you want, but you'll need to follow some rules about what you eat.

The renal diet can be used by anyone, regardless of their health status or age. People who follow this diet must know how to take care of themselves, so they don't have any complications.

How Much Protein Intake?

Understand how much protein is important: current recommendations suggest that people with chronic kidney disease should consume a minimum of 0.8g/kg per day, and for patients on Dialysis, proteins are maintained between 1-1.2g/kg/day.

Keep track of your fluid intake: adequate fluid intake helps compensate for losses in blood volume. If you have diabetes, your doctor will commend an additional 8 ounces of fluid each day.

Avoid stress: stress can lead to symptoms similar to hypertension, dry skin, high blood pressure, and fatigue. If you notice any changes in your kidney function, including daytime fatigue, you should consult your doctor immediately.

Don't obsess about how much protein you eat: people with chronic kidney disease often obsess about protein intake because they find it hard to digest protein; however, this is not necessary. Most available protein is digested without problems by people with chronic kidney disease. It also doesn't matter what form of protein you consume — animal or plant-based — as long as it carries all nine essential amino acids. Try incorporating more legumes into your diets, such as lentils, beans, and chickpeas. People with chronic kidney disease almost completely digest legumes without negative consequences.

Is Fish Good for the Kidney?

Some studies have shown that fish (especially fatty fish) is suitable for chronic kidney disease people. These studies have looked at how much fat (or saturated fat) people should eat and provide information about how to prepare and cook fish. Many experts believe that a diet low in protein (especially animal protein) may help chronic kidney disease. Some experts suggest avoiding foods that contain MSG or high levels of sodium chloride (salt) – especially if you have a record of heart failure or stroke.

Tips to Manage Chronic Kidney Disease

According to studies, following a renal diet can control many of the symptoms associated with this illness, such as fatigue, increased urination, and dizziness. Therefore, if you have chronic kidney disease, it may be good to follow a renal diet if you suffer from these symptoms.

Choose Well-Balanced Meals

This is naturally the best way to manage chronic kidney disease. If your diet is predominantly high in salt, fat, and protein — which is what you would expect if you have dyslipidemia — you will probably end up with recurring symptoms of chronic kidney disease that could eventually guide to dialysis treatment. Don't cut down on calories too much! Many people with chronic kidney disease restrict their food intake to lose weight, making it harder for them to control their heart rate and blood pressure. By eating well-balanced meals, you will also help prevent the growth of new kidney stones. Many people with chronic kidney disease restrict their food intake to lose weight, making it harder for them to control their heart rate and blood pressure. By eating well-balanced meals, you will also help prevent the growth of new kidney stones. Avoid late evening snacks! Eat a small amount of food early in the day or make a quick snack before dinner instead of eating late at night when most people feel like having junk food.

Eat Smart

Eat a small amount of food early in the day or make a quick snack before dinner instead of eating late at night when most people feel like having junk food.

Eat Frozen or... Canned

This may seem like news to you, but fruit, when frozen or canned, tends to retain more of its nutrients, as the product is frozen or canned at its peak. The only thing you need to keep in mind is to choose products that have no added salt or, in the case of fruit, that the percentage is 100%.

Slow Cook Is the Answer

You should start using a slow cooker. The latter allows you to make tender protein just by starting with frozen chicken. Try it for yourself. Plus, you can make it in large quantities, divide it into single-serving containers, and store it in the freezer. You can use it as an accompaniment to your dishes.

Grocery Shopping

Be smart when you go grocery shopping. Before you leave the house, be sure to check what you already have in your fridge and make a detailed list of everything you'll need, so you know exactly what to buy and don't waste time. Also, more importantly, make sure you don't go hungry. This way, you'll avoid putting foods in your cart that you can't eat.

Bad Habits to Avoid

The causes of CKD include genetics and bad habits. A few examples of bad habits include Smoking cigarettes, lack of exercise, obesity, and high blood pressure. Genetics also plays a role. For example, people of African descent are at a higher risk for having CKD. If you have a parent or grandparent with a CKD family history, you are also at a higher risk. If you or a family is agonizing from the effects of chronic kidney disease (CKD), you may be wondering what lifestyle changes can be made to minimize the impact on your life.

As you know, kidney disease is a progressive condition that can result in much longer-term consequences than you might originally anticipate. Fortunately, you can make numerous lifestyle changes to minimize the impact of CKD on your life.

Aside from reducing salt intake, there are several other strategies that you can use to manage CKD and its progression. For instance, smoking is associated with an increased risk of developing CKD and other health conditions. Thus, if you're trying to prevent the onset of CKD, consider quitting smoking for good. Other lifestyle changes to consider include eating more fruits and vegetables, getting more physical activity, and following a high-fiber diet.

What to Do to Eat Right During Kidney Disease

Keep Your Sodium in Check

One of kidney disease's patients is to keep blood pressure under control; it is crucial not to overdo sodium intake. The ideal amount of sodium for patients suffering from kidney disease is less than 2,300 milligrams per day.

So how can you avoid taking in too much sodium? Below you'll find several very helpful tips.

- Avoid frozen or canned foods that contain too much sodium
- Learn to read nutritional labels on convenience foods (if the percentage of sodium is equal to or more than 20%, it means that the amount of sodium is too high; in other words, a percent daily value equal to or less than 5% will mean that that food is low in sodium)
- Buy fresh foods and cook them; this will allow you to regulate your sodium intake
- use spices instead of salt
- if you buy canned foods, be sure to rinse them well before consumption, as the preserving liquid usually contains a lot of salt.

Keep Your Heart Healthy

For patients suffering from kidney disease, it is crucial to choose healthy foods not only for the kidneys but also for the heart.

It is essential to prevent the fat present in foods from accumulating in the blood vessels and the kidneys.

To prevent this from happening, you can, for example, eliminate fat from meat before cooking it or avoid foods that contain an excessive amount of saturated fat (just read the nutritional labels).

You can also use tricks not only in the choice of foods but also in the way you decide to cook them. Therefore, it is preferable to use grilling, baking, broiling, stir-frying instead of deep-frying. Or use cooking spray to moisten pans instead of using butter.

29

Less alcohol is better

Also, it is important to limit alcohol. If you are a woman, no more than one drink per day; if you are a man, no more than two drinks per day.

In any case, it's always best to let a dietitian help you know exactly how much alcohol you can or cannot take.

Understanding Nutrition During CKD

Protein

If you've heard that for CKD patients, protein is bad for them, you need to know that's not the case.

Renal diet does not eliminate proteins; Protein is one of the fundamental macronutrients in a person's diet, and there are both animal and vegetable sources.

However, it is also true that in CKD patients, protein intake should vary depending on the level of kidney function, body size, and other factors. In general, they are well maintained at 0.8g/kg per day as the maximum amount in CKD, and for patients on dialysis, proteins are maintained between 1-1.2g/kg/day.

Therefore, your nutritionist must guide you in defining the correct protein intake to include in your diet.

In any case, below, you will find a table with the best protein sources in terms of quality.

Vegetables	Legumes	Egg & Soy	Dairy*	Cereals	Poultry Meat & Seafood**
Carrots	Peas, green,	Edamame	Yoghurt, plain	Oatmeal	Chicken
Coleslaw	canned	Tofu	Milk, whole	Rice	Lamb
Eggplant	Beans	Eggs, egg white	and fat-free	Wheat	Turkey
Lettuce	Lentils		Cheese	Unsalted	Fish
Broccoli			(cheddar,	crackers	Shrimp
Cabbage, green			mozzarella,	Pasta	Tuna
and red			swiss)	Tortilla	
Celery			ice-cream	Bread	
Cauliflower			Cottage cheese	Bun	
Cucumbers			Custard	(hamburger)	

Best Protein Sources

* 1 serving = ½ cup of milk or yogurt, or one slice of cheese
** 1 cooked serving = 2 to 3 ounces

Potassium

Checking that your blood potassium level is not too high or too low is necessary to let your nerves and muscles work the right way.

However, it is not easy to know when your blood potassium level is too high. For this reason, your healthcare provider will be the one who needs to take this measurement. In general, your blood potassium level should be between 3.5 and 5.0.

But how do you reduce your blood potassium level? Here are some steps:

- Use spices and herbs instead of salt.
- drain canned fruits and vegetables before consuming them
- eat smaller portions of high-protein foods
- eat fruits and vegetables with the low potassium content

For example, it is preferable to eat white rice instead of brown rice; or white bread instead of brown bread; rice milk instead of cow's late.

Low Potassium Fruits & Vegetables (200 mg or less)

Fruits	Vegetables
• Apples	• Eggplants
• Peaches	• Bell peppers
• Apricots (canned)	• Kales
• Plums	• Broccoli (fresh)
• Berries	• Green beans
• Cranberry juice	• Cabbage
• Pineapple	• Mushrooms (fresh)
• Grapes	• Carrots
• Tangerines	• Celery
• Lemons and limes	• Cauliflowers
• Watermelon	• Onions
• Mangos	• Cucumber
• Papayas	• Corn
• Pears	• Lettuce

Hight Potassium Fruits & Vegetables (More than 200 mg)

Fruits	Vegetables
• Bananas	• Tomatoes / tomato sauce
• Raisins	• Avocado
• Cantaloupe	• Sweet potatoes
• Oranges / orange juice	• Baked beans
• Nectarines	• Lentils, beans
• Kiwi	• Broccoli (cooked)
• Prunes / prune juice	• Spinach (cooked)
• Apricots (fresh)	• Brussel sprouts (cooked)
	• Pumpkin
	• Chard
	• Potatoes
	• Chile peppers
	• Mushrooms (cooked)

Phosphorus

For each of us, phosphorus represents a fundamental component of our body because it contributes to maintaining bone health.

However, for people who suffer from chronic kidney disease, phosphorus tends to accumulate in the bloodstream, which has the opposite effect of making bones weaker and causing joint pain.

It is for this reason that CKD patients should take foods that are low in phosphorus.

Remember that the ideal phosphorus intake per day should be between 800 and 1000 milligrams.

Where is the Phosphorus Contained?

Foods Higher in Phosphorus	Foods Lower in Phosphorus
• Meat*	• Vegetables
• Poultry*	• Fresh fruit
• Fish*	• Pasta
• Beans**	• Rice
• Lentils**	• Bread
• Nuts***	• Rice cereals
• Dairy foods****	• Corn
• Bran cereals	
• Oatmeal	

*1 cooked serving= 2 to 3 ounces
**1 serving = ½ cup cooked beans or lentils
***1 serving = ¼ cup
****1 serving = ½ cup of milk or yogurt

Sodium

To understand what sodium is, you need only think of salt. One teaspoon of salt? As much as 2300 milligrams of sodium. You wouldn't have guessed that, would you?

In general, we should all decrease our salt intake, which would allow us to reduce the risk of increasing blood pressure or developing cardiovascular disease.

Especially in patients with chronic kidney disease, sodium is a sensitive issue. Their kidneys can no longer balance sodium and water in the body, which causes an increase in blood pressure.

In patients with CKD, sodium intake should be less than 1500 mg per day.

But how can you tell where the sodium is? In addition to the list below with high and low sodium foods, there are a few tricks you can follow to immediately identify where sodium is contained and where it's not:

- always read the nutritional labels of foods to choose foods that have a percentage of average value equal to 5% or less (if it is equal to or exceeds 20%, the rate is high)
- buy foods that have the words: sodium-free, salt-free, low sodium, very low sodium, unsalted
- be careful with fresh meat; sodium may have been added to help preserve the meat

Where is the Sodium Contained?

Foods Higher in Sodium	Foods Lower in Sodium
• Low- fat, low-sodium cheese	• Ready-to-eat foods
• Fresh Meat	• Bacon, ham, hot dogs, sausage
• Fresh Poultry	• Olives, pickles, relish
• Fresh Fish	• Canned beans, chicken, meat and fish
• Rice	• Pretzels, chips, salted nuts
• Cooked cereals without added salt	• Salt and salt seasonings
• Fresh fruit	• Canned vegetables
• Frozen Fruit	• Frozen meals
• Fresh vegetables	• Cottage cheese
• Frozen vegetables	• Canned tomato products
• Unsalted nuts	• Soy sauce

In conclusion, then, to avoid consuming too much sodium, the best tips are:

- cook fresh food and avoid ready-made meals
- replace salt with aromatic herbs, spices, and low-sodium condiments
- rinse well vegetables, meat, fish, and canned legumes

Four Weeks Meal Plan

First Week

Day	Breakfast	Lunch	Dinner
Day-1	Tropical Oatmeal	Chicken and Mushroom Stew	Healthy Steamed Fish
Day-2	Sourdough Pancakes	Roasted Carrot Soup	Broiled Salmon in Maple
Day-3	Overnight Oats	Garlic and Butter-Flavored Cod	Chickpea Curry and Eggplant
Day-4	Coconut Pancakes	Healthy Tilapia Broccoli Platter	Chickpea Bites and Eggplant
Day-5	Kidney-Friendly Breakfast Burrito	Parsley Scallops	Sesame Asparagus
Day-6	Cranberry and Oatmeal Breakfast Cookies	Blackened Chicken	Rosemary and Roasted Cauliflower
Day-7	Breakfast Eggs with Tortilla	Spicy Paprika Lamb Chops	Green Bean Garlic Salad

Second Week

Day	Breakfast	Lunch	Dinner
Day-8	Bread and Sausage Breakfast Casserole	Healthy Mushroom and Olive Sirloin Steak	Shrimp Spaghetti
Day-9	Apple Oatmeal Crisp	Healthy Parsley and Chicken Breast	Pork Pineapple Roast
Day-10	Apple Oatmeal Custard	Simple Mustard Chicken	Curry Pork Lime Kebabs
Day-11	Texas Toast Casserole	Healthy Golden Eggplant Fries	Beef Salad
Day-12	Zucchini Bread	Very Wild Mushroom Pilaf	Chicken Stew with Kale and Mushrooms
Day-13	Garlic Mayo Bread	Sporty Baby Carrots	Healthy Rice and Chicken Soup
Day-14	Chia Pudding	Saucy Garlic Greens	Healthy Panini

Third Week

Day	Breakfast	Lunch	Dinner
Day-15	Parmesan Zucchini Frittata	Garden Salad	Chicken Sandwich
Day-16	Apple Cinnamon Rings	Spicy Cabbage Dish	Tomato stuffed Portobello Caps
Day-17	Yogurt Bulgur	Extreme Balsamic Chicken	Swordfish and Citrus Salsa Delight
Day-18	Deviled Eggs	Enjoyable Green lettuce and Bean Medley	Roasted Halibut with Banana-Orange Relish
Day-19	Cream Cheese Omelet	Low Caloric Cauliflower and Dill Mash	Salad Greens with Roasted Beets
Day-20	Breakfast Potato Latkes with Spinach	Peas Soup	Maple Glazed Steak
Day-21	Easy Turnip Puree	Cauliflower Rice and Coconut	Bavarian Pot Roast

Fourth Week

Day	Breakfast	Lunch	Dinner
Day-22	Green lettuce Bacon Breakfast Bake	Kale and Garlic Platter	Black Bean Burger and Cilantro Slaw
Day-23	Healthy Green lettuce Tomato Muffins	Blistered Beans and Almond	BBQ Ribs with Marinade
Day-24	Chicken Egg Breakfast Muffin	Cucumber Soup	Herb Crusted Roast Leg of Lamb
Day-25	Breakfast Egg Salad	Eggplant Salad	Curried Turkey with Rice
Day-26	Vegetable Tofu Scramble	Cajun Crab	Feta and Spinach Pita Bake
Day-27	Cheese Coconut Pancake	Mushroom Pork Chops	Chili Con Carne with Rice
Day-28	Cheesy Scrambled Eggs with Fresh Herbs	Caramelized Pork Chops	Marinated Shrimp

Breakfast

1. Tropical Oatmeal

Preparation Time: 5 minutes

Cooking Time: 13 minutes

Servings: 4 (2/3 cup per servings)

Ingredients:

- 1 cup uncooked rolled oats
- 1 1/4 cups coconut milk beverage (or other vegetable drink)
- 1 1/2 tablespoons chia seeds
- 1 mango (medium sized fruit), peeled, seeded, and cubed
- 1/4 cup unsweetened coconut flakes

Directions:

1. Take a saucepan and cook the oats along with the light coconut milk (or other vegetable drink if you prefer) and chia seeds over medium-high heat.
2. As soon as it starts to boil, turn down the heat and leave for another 10 minutes. The liquid should absorb completely.
3. Grab four bowls and divide. Garnish with coconut flakes and diced mango.

Nutrition Facts Per Serving:

Total Fat: 14.2 g
Cholesterol: 0 mg
Sodium: 34.6 mg
Total Carbohydrate: 50.1 g
Dietary Fiber: 9.4 g
Protein: 8.6 g
Potassium: 350 mg
Phosphorus: 278.6 mg

2. Sourdough Pancakes

Preparation Time: 5 minutes

Cooking Time: 8 minutes

Servings: 2

Ingredients:

- 2 medium-sized eggs
- 2 cups sourdough starter
- 1 tablespoon honey

- 0.25 teaspoon baking soda

Directions:

1. First, crack the eggs, separate the whites from the yolks, and place them in two separate bowls.
2. Next, lightly beat the yolks and also the egg whites, making sure to wash the whips well. At this point, add honey to the egg whites and the sourdough starter in the yolks.
3. Then, gently incorporate the egg whites into the yolks and add the baking soda into the batter that has formed.
4. At this point, cook the pancakes on a well-greased skillet over medium-high heat. When bubbles appear on the surface, flip the pancake over and cook it on the other side.

Nutrition Facts Per Serving:

Calories: 519 Kcal
Sodium: 63 mg
Total Carbohydrate: 82g
Protein: 23 g
Potassium: 43 mg
Phosphorus: 113 mg

3. Overnight Oats

Preparation Time: 5 minutes

Cooking Time: 5 minutes

Servings: 4

Ingredients:

- 3/4 cup rolled oats
- 1/2 cup canned coconut milk
- 3/4 cup unsweetened almond milk
- 1 tablespoon chia seeds
- 1/4 teaspoon ground cinnamon (optional)

Directions:

1. Take a glass bowl with an airtight seal (even a simple container with a good lid will do) and combine all

the ingredients, taking care to mix them well to blend the flavors well.

2. After sealing the glass bowl (or container), place it in the refrigerator and let it sit overnight (if you're short on time, leave it in the fridge for at least 8 hours).

3. The following day, or after at least 8 hours have passed, serve in bowls and garnish with berries, nuts, coconut flakes, or seeds.

Nutrition Facts Per Serving:

Total Fat: 15.1 g
Cholesterol: 0 mg
Sodium: 78.1 mg
Total Carbohydrates: 25.1 g
Dietary Fiber: 5.2 g
Protein: 6.5 g
Iron: 3.8 mg
Potassium: 610.3 mg
Phosphorus: 232.5 mg

4. Coconut Pancakes

Preparation Time: 5 minutes

Cooking Time: 8 minutes

Servings: 2

Ingredients:

- 1/2 cup + 2 tablespoons all-purpose flour
- 1 1/2 tablespoons granulated brown sugar (or honey, if preferred)
- 1/2 teaspoon baking soda
- 1 teaspoon cream of tartar
- 1/4 cup canned coconut milk
- 1/2 teaspoon coconut oil
- 2–4 tablespoons water (more or less for thick but pourable consistency)
- 1/4 teaspoon vanilla or coconut extract

For the Toppings:

- 1 1/4 tablespoons maple syrup
- 1/4 cup unsweetened coconut flakes
- 1/2 cup canned pineapple, drained

Directions:

1. First, take a bowl and combine all the dry ingredients, i.e., flour, sugar, baking soda, and cream of tartar, and mix.
2. At this point, combine the liquid ingredients, namely coconut oil, coconut milk, water, vanilla extract, or coconut extract, taking care to beat the mixture well to prevent lumps from forming.
3. If necessary, add more water and continue to blend.
4. Now, heat a cast-iron skillet over medium-high heat with a drizzle of coconut oil. As soon as the pan is hot, pour in 1/4 cup of batter at a time and let it cook for about 3-5 minutes until the first bubbles appear.
5. At that point, flip the pancake over and let it cook on the other side for another 3 minutes.
6. Serve with desired toppings.

Nutrition Facts Per Serving:

Calories: 388.25 Kcal
Total Fat: 17.26 g
Carbs: 56.47 g
Sugars: 26.16 g
Fiber: 3.24 g
Cholesterol: 0 mg
Sodium: 12.16 mg
Total Carbohydrate: 56.47 g
Dietary Fiber: 3.24 g
Protein: 4.95 g
Potassium: 366.5 mg
Phosphorus: 114 mg

5. Fluffy Mock Pancakes

Preparation Time: 5 minutes
Cooking Time: 10 minutes
Servings: 2

Ingredients:

- 1 egg
- 1 cup ricotta cheese
- 1 teaspoon cinnamon

- 2 tablespoons honey, add more if needed

Directions:

1. Using a blender, put together egg, honey, cinnamon, and ricotta cheese. Process until all ingredients are well combined.
2. Pour an equal amount of the blended mixture into the pan. Cook each pancake for 4 minutes on both sides. Serve.

Nutrition Facts Per Serving:

Calories: 188.1 kcal
Total Fat: 14.5 g
Saturated Fat: 4.5 g
Cholesterol: 139.5 mg
Sodium: 175.5 mg
Total Carbs: 5.5 g
Fiber: 2.8 g
Sugar: 0.9 g
Protein: 8.5 g

6. Spicy Veggie Pancakes

Preparation Time: 10 minutes
Cooking Time: 20 minutes
Servings: 4

Ingredients:

- 3 tbsp. olive oil, divided
- 2 small onions, finely chopped
- 1 jalapeño pepper, minced
- 3/4 cup carrot, grated
- 3/4 cup cabbage, finely chopped
- 1 cup quick-cooking oats
- 3/4 cup water
- 1/2 cup whole-wheat flour
- 1 large egg white
- 0.5 tsp. baking soda
- 1/4 tsp. cayenne pepper

Directions:

1. Take a large skillet and heat 2 tsp. oil over medium heat.

2. Sauté the onion, jalapeño, carrot, and cabbage for 4 minutes.
3. While the veggies are cooking, mix the oats, rice, water, flour, egg white, baking soda, and cayenne pepper in a medium bowl.
4. Then, add the cooked vegetables to the mixture and stir to combine.
5. Heat the remaining oil in a large skillet over medium heat.
6. Drop the mixture into the skillet, about 1/3 cup per pancake. Cook for 4 minutes, or until bubbles form on the pancakes' surface and the edges look cooked, then carefully flip them over.
7. Repeat with the remaining mixture and serve.

Nutrition Facts Per Serving:

Calories: 529.08 kcal
Total Fat: 24.96 g
Carbs: 68.28 g

Protein: 12.08 g
Sodium: 71.45 mg
Potassium: 600 mg
Phosphorus: 320 mg

7. Mock Cream Cheese Pancake

Preparation time: 5 minutes

Cooking time: 5 minutes

Servings: 4

Ingredients:

- 1 pack Stevia
- 1/2 tsp. cinnamon
- 2 eggs
- 1 cup cream cheese

Directions:

1. Put eggs, cream cheese, Stevia, and cinnamon in a blender. Processes until all ingredients are well-combined.
2. Pour an equal amount of the blended mixture in a greased pan. Cook for 4 minutes on both sides. Repeat with the rest of the batter. Serve.

Nutrition Facts Per Serving:

Calories 289.6 kcal
Protein 13.16 g
Potassium 199 mg
Sodium: 82 mg
Carbs: 2.5 g
Fat: 26.6 g
Phosphorus: 282.7 mg

8. Kidney-friendly Breakfast Burrito

Preparation Time: 5 minutes
Cooking Time: 5 minutes
Servings: 2

Ingredients:

- 4 eggs
- 3 tablespoons Ortega green Chiles, diced
- 1/4 teaspoon ground cumin
- 1/2 teaspoon hot pepper sauce
- 2 flour tortillas, burrito size
- Non-stick cooking spray

Directions:

1. First, take a bowl and whisk the eggs together with the hot sauce, cumin, and green chiles.
2. At this point, pour the mixture into a medium-sized non-stick skillet, previously heated with cooking spray, and cook for 3-4 minutes.
3. Meanwhile, place the tortillas in the microwave and heat them for about 20 seconds (if you don't have a microwave, you can heat the tortillas in a hot skillet).
4. Divide the mixture between the two tortillas and roll up to form a burrito.

Nutrition Facts Per Serving:

Calories: 220 kcal
Total Fat: 18 g
Cholesterol: 372 mg
Sodium: 594 mg
Total Carbohydrate: 33 g

Dietary Fiber: 2.5 g

Protein: 11 g

Potassium: 175 mg

Phosphorus: 182 mg

9. Cranberry and Oatmeal Breakfast Cookies

Preparation Time: 5 minutes

Cooking Time: 15 minutes

Servings: 4

Ingredients:

- 2 oz. unsalted butter
- 2 tablespoons granulated brown sugar or stevia
- 1 large egg
- 1/4 cup all-purpose flour
- 1/4 teaspoon salt
- 1/2 teaspoon cinnamon
- 1 teaspoon vanilla extract
- 1 oz. vanilla whey protein powder
- 1 cup applesauce
- 1/2 cup dried cranberries
- 2 cups rolled oats

Directions:

1. Start by preheating the oven to 350 F and lining a baking sheet with parchment paper.
2. Next, soften the butter and mix it with the sugar or stevia using an electric mixer, and next, add the egg, flour, vanilla extract, protein powder, salt, and cinnamon. Mix well and then add the applesauce and mix again.
3. At this point, pour in the cranberries and oats and mix the mixture well.
4. Take the baking sheet and spread 1/4 cup scoop of the mixture, and flatten each cookie. Let bake in the preheated oven until golden brown.
5. Once baked, let the cookies cool for at least 5 minutes on the baking sheet and only then transfer them to a rack or plate.

Calories: 810.37 kcal

Total Fat: 34.9 g

Cholesterol: 43 mg

Sodium: 385.69 mg

Total Carbohydrate: 148.7 g

Sugars: 59.5 g

Dietary Fiber: 2.6 g

Protein: 24.66 g

Potassium: 966.43 mg

Phosphorus: 841.32 mg

10. Breakfast Eggs with Tortilla

Preparation Time: 5 minutes

Cooking Time: 5 minutes

Servings: 2

Ingredients:

- 1 corn tortilla, 6" size
- 2 whole eggs
- 2 egg whites
- 3 green onions, chopped
- 2 slices tomato, each slice 1/4" thick, chopped
- 2 tablespoons canola oil

Directions:

1. Heat corn tortilla in the microwave for 2 minutes maximum.
2. Once ready, cut the tortilla into small pieces and shape them into chips.
3. At this point, take a bowl and whisk together the eggs with the egg whites, and set them aside.
4. Now, take a frying pan, heat the oil over medium heat, and sauté the onions for about 1 minute.
5. Next, add the egg and egg white mixture, tomato, and tortillas and stir until the eggs are set.

Nutrition Facts Per Serving:

Calories: 230 kcal

Total Fat: 19 g

Cholesterol: 165 mg

Sodium: 115 mg

Total Carbohydrate: 9 g

Dietary Fiber: 1.3 g

Protein: 11 g
Potassium: 222 mg
Phosphorus: 147 mg

11. Bread and Sausage Breakfast Casserole

Preparation Time: 5 minutes

Cooking Time: 55 minutes

Servings: 4

Ingredients:

- 8 ounces reduced-fat pork sausage
- 8 ounces cream cheese
- 1 cup 1% low-fat milk
- 5 large eggs
- 1/2 teaspoon dry mustard
- 1/2 teaspoon dried onion flakes
- 4 slices white bread, cubed or broken

Directions:

1. First, preheat the oven to 325 F.
2. Next, heat a medium skillet and cook the sausage. Once ready, set aside.
3. At this point, in a blender, pour all the other ingredients, except for the bread, and blend. Then add the cooked sausage and continue to mix until the mixture is homogeneous.
4. Now, take the bread that we didn't use before and place it on a greased 9" x 9" casserole dish. Pour the sausage mixture over the bread and bake for 55 minutes or until fully cooked.

Nutrition Facts Per Serving:

Calories: 484.77 kcal
Total Fat: 31.42 g
Cholesterol: 149 mg
Sodium: 721.3 mg
Total Carbohydrate: 24.24 g
Dietary Fiber: 0.4 g
Protein: 26.45 g
Potassium: 441.52 mg
Phosphorus: 347.89 mg

12. Apple Oatmeal Crisp

Preparation Time: 5 minutes

Cooking Time: 35 minutes

Servings: 2

Ingredients:

- 1 cup whole oatmeal
- 1/2 cup all-purpose flour
- 3/4 cup brown sugar
- 1 teaspoon cinnamon
- 3 tbsp butter
- 3 Granny Smith apples

Directions:

1. First, preheat the oven to 350 F.
2. Take a medium-sized bowl and combine the oatmeal with brown sugar, all-purpose flour, and cinnamon.
3. At this point, cut the butter (you can help yourself with a pastry cutter) and add it to the mixture, taking care to mix the whole mixture well.
4. Arrange the sliced apples on a 9 x 9 baking sheet and pour the mixture on top. Bake for 30-35 minutes.

Nutrition Facts Per Serving:

Calories: 784.69 kcal

Total Fat: 13 g

Cholesterol: 32 mg

Sodium: 95 mg

Total Carbohydrate: 42 g

Dietary Fiber: 2.4 g

Protein: 3 g

Potassium: 560 mg

Phosphorus: 210 mg

13. Apple Oatmeal Custard

Preparation Time: 5 minutes

Cooking Time: 3 minutes

Servings: 2

Ingredients:

- 1/3 cup quick-cooking oatmeal
- 1 large egg
- 1/2 cup almond milk

- 1/4 teaspoon cinnamon
- 1/2 medium apple, cored and finely chopped

Directions:

1. Take a relatively large bowl and combine the oatmeal with the egg and almond milk. Help yourself with a fork to mix well, and afterward, add the cinnamon and apple and mix again, making sure to blend well.
2. Cook the mixture in the microwave for 2 minutes at maximum temperature and then remove from the microwave and stir again. If necessary, let it cook for another 30-60 seconds.
3. If the consistency is too thick, add a little more milk or water.

Nutrition Facts Per Serving:

Calories 330 kcal
Total Fat: 8 g
Cholesterol: 186 mg

Sodium: 164 mg
Total Carbohydrate: 33 g
Dietary Fiber: 5.8 g
Protein: 11 g
Potassium: 362 mg
Phosphorus: 240 mg

14. Texas Toast Casserole

Preparation Time: 10 minutes

Cooking Time: 30 minutes

Servings: 10

Ingredients:

- 1/2 cup butter, melted
- 1 cup brown Swerve
- 0.25 lb. Texas Toast bread, sliced
- 4 large eggs
- 1 1/2 cup milk
- 1 tbsp. vanilla extract
- 2 tbsps. Swerve
- 2 tsps. cinnamon
- 2 tbsp. Maple syrup for serving

Directions:

1. First, take a 9x13-inch baking dish, coat it with

53

cooking spray and arrange the bread slices on top.

2. In a mixer, combine the eggs and all the other ingredients and mix everything until smooth and even.
3. Pour the mixture over the bread slices and bake in the preheated oven for 30 minutes at 370 F.
4. Serve with maple syrup.

Nutrition Facts Per Serving:

Calories: 332 kcal
Total Fat: 13.7 g
Saturated Fat: 6.9 g
Cholesterol: 102 mg
Sodium: 280 mg
Carbohydrates: 50 g
Dietary Fiber: 2 g
Sugars: 4 g
Protein: 7.4 g
Calcium: 143 mg
Phosphorus: 186 mg
Potassium: 74 mg

15. Breakfast Cheesecake

Preparation time: 5 minutes

Cooking time: 15 minutes

Servings: 16

Ingredients:

- 1/2 cup uncured sausage
- 2 tbsps. honey
- 2 cups cottage cheese
- Pepper, 1/4 tsp.
- 1/2 tsp. olive oil
- 3 cups Greek yogurt
- Salt, 1/4 tsp.
- 4 eggs
- 2 tsps. vanilla
- 1/2 chopped onion

Directions:

1. In a blender, combine eggs, cream cheese, cottage cheese, honey, and vanilla. Processes until all ingredients are well combined.
2. Meanwhile, warm the olive oil in a pan. Saute onion and uncured sausage. Season with salt

54

and pepper. Cook for 4 minutes. Transfer the mixture into a baking dish.

3. Set inside the oven and bake for 10 minutes. Allow to cool at room temperature. Refrigerate for 1 hour before serving.

Nutrition Facts Per Serving:

Calories: 1228.56 kcal
Total Fat: 63.53 g
Carbs: 57.38 g
Sugars: 53.28 g
Protein: 103.71 g
Sodium: 1200.23 mg
Potassium: 500 mg
Phosphorus: 350 mg

16. Zucchini Bread

Preparation Time: 10 minutes

Cooking Time: 1 hour

Servings: 16

Ingredients:

- 2 eggs
- 1/2 cup Swerve
- 1 cup apple sauce
- 2 cups zucchini, shredded
- 1 tsp. vanilla
- 2 cups flour
- 1/4 tsp. baking powder
- 1 tsp. baking soda
- 1 tsp. cinnamon
- 1/2 tsp. ginger
- 0.5 cup unsalted nuts, chopped

Directions:

1. First, preheat the oven to 375 F.
2. Take a large bowl and combine the eggs, zucchini, applesauce and the rest of the ingredients, mix well until evenly combined.
3. Once you have the desired consistency, spread the mixture onto a 13 x 9 baking dish and bake for 1 hour at 375 F.
4. Finally, cut into slices and serve.

Calories: 700.78 kcal

Total Fat: 4.79 g

Saturated Fat: 0.9 g

Cholesterol: 31 mg

Sodium: 21.36 mg

Carbohydrates: 34.91 g

Dietary Fiber: 1.6 g

Sugars: 2.99 g

Protein: 4.12 g

Calcium: 20 mg

Phosphorus: 55 mg

Potassium: 98.59 mg

17. Garlic Mayo Bread

Preparation Time: 10 minutes

Cooking Time: 5 minutes

Servings: 16

Ingredients:

- 3 tbsps. vegetable oil
- 4 cloves garlic, minced
- 2 tsp. Paprika Dash cayenne pepper
- 1 tsp. lemon juice
- 2 tbsp. cheddar cheese, grated
- 3/4 cup lite mayonnaise
- 0.25 lb. loaf French bread, sliced
- 1 tsp. Italian herbs

Directions:

1. First, take a small bowl and combine the garlic with the oil and let them marinate together overnight.
2. Afterward, remove the garlic and keep only the oil, which will have a strong garlic aroma at this point.
3. At this point, combine the flavored garlic oil with cayenne, paprika, lemon juice, mayonnaise, and cheddar.
4. Prepare a baking sheet lined with parchment paper and lay the bread slices on it and the mayonnaise mixture and Italian herbs on top.

5. Bake the bread slices in a hot oven for 5 minutes and serve.

Calories: 594.19 kcal
Total Fat: 34.08 g
Saturated Fat: 1.8 g
Cholesterol: 5 mg
Sodium: 423 mg
Carbohydrates: 60.42 g
Dietary Fiber: 1.3 g
Sugars: 2 g
Protein 11.68 g
Calcium: 56 mg
Phosphorus: 230.09 mg
Potassium: 272.39 mg

18.   Chia Pudding

Preparation Time: 10 minutes
Cooking Time: 0 minutes
Servings: 2

Ingredients:

- 1/2 cup raspberries
- 2 tsp. maple syrup
- 1 1/2 cup Plain yogurt
- 1/4 tsp. ground cardamom
- 1/3 cup Chia seeds, dried

Directions:

1. Take a bowl and combine the plain yogurt with maple syrup and ground cardamom. Finish with the chia seeds and mix well.
2. Take serving glasses and arrange the yogurt mixture inside and garnish with the raspberries.
3. Let sit in the fridge for at least 30 minutes or even overnight.

Nutrition Facts Per Serving:

Calories: 303 kcal
Fat: 16 g
Fiber: 11.8 g
Carbs: 33.2 g
Protein: 15.5 g
Phosphorus: 470 mg
Potassium: 460 mg

19. Parmesan Zucchini Frittata

Preparation Time: 10 minutes

Cooking Time: 35 minutes

Servings: 6

Ingredients:

- 1 tbsp. olive oil
- 1 cup yellow onion, sliced
- 3 cups zucchini, chopped
- 1/2 cup Cheddar cheese, grated
- 5 large eggs
- 1/2 tsp. black pepper
- 1/8 tsp. paprika
- 3 tbsp. parsley, chopped

Directions:

1. Take a large bowl and combine the shredded zucchini with the onion, parsley, eggs, and other ingredients. Mix well and pour the mixture onto an 11x7 inch baking dish, unforming it well.
2. Bake and let bake for about 35 minutes at 350 F.
3. Once ready, cut into slices and serve.

Nutrition Facts Per Serving:

Calories: 440 kcal

Total Fat: 9.7 g

Saturated Fat: 2.8 g

Cholesterol: 250 mg

Sodium: 123 mg

Carbohydrates: 4.7 g

Protein: 8 g

Phosphorus: 166 mg

Potassium: 280 mg

20. Apple Cinnamon Rings

Preparation Time: 10 minutes

Cooking Time: 20 minutes

Servings: 6

Ingredients:

- 4 large apples cut in rings
- 1 cup flour
- 1/4 tsp. baking powder
- 1/4 tsp. cinnamon
- 1 large egg, beaten
- 1 cup 1% fat milk

- Vegetable oil, for frying

Cinnamon Topping:

- 1/3 cup of brown Swerve
- 2 tsps. cinnamon

Directions:

1. Take a bowl and combine the flour with the baking powder and cinnamon and mix well.
2. Separately, beat the egg with the milk in another bowl and then pour it into the dry flour mixture. Mix the mixture well until the batter is smooth and even.
3. At this point, heat oil in a wok until 375 F.
4. Then, dip the apple rings into the batter and then lay it in the wok, and fry it until golden brown.
5. Once cooked, transfer the apple rings to a tray lined with paper towels.
6. Garnish with cinnamon and Swerve as topping and serve.

Nutrition Facts Per Serving:

Calories: 166 kcal

Total Fat: 1.7 g

Saturated Fat: 0.5 g

Cholesterol: 33 mg

Sodium: 55 mg

Carbohydrates: 13.1 g

Sugars: 14 g

Protein: 4.7 g

Phosphorus: 97 mg

Potassium: 208 mg

21. Yogurt Bulgur

Preparation Time: 10 minutes

Cooking Time: 18 minutes

Servings: 3

Ingredients:

- 1 cup bulgur
- 1 1/2 cup water
- 1/2 tsp. salt
- 1 tsp. olive oil
- 2 cups Greek plain yogurt

Directions:

1. First, take a medium-sized saucepan and heat the oil

over medium heat. Then, lay the bulgur on top of the casserole dish and let it roast, still over medium heat, for 2-3 minutes, making sure to occasionally move the bulgur around, so it doesn't burn.

2. At this point, add the water and salt, close the lid and let it cook for another 15 minutes over medium heat.

3. Once the bulgur is cooked, let it cool, add it to the Greek yogurt and mix well. Transfer to serving plates and serve well chilled.

Nutrition Facts Per Serving:

Calories: 301.98 kcal

Fat: 8.86 g

Fiber: 5.8 g

Carbs: 40.51 g

Protein: 19.2 g

Sodium: 444.55 mg

Potassium: 362 mg

Phosphorus: 240 mg

22. Deviled Eggs

Preparation Time: 5 minutes

Cooking Time: 8 minutes

Servings: 2

Ingredients:

- 4 eggs
- 1 tbsp. chopped onion
- 1/2 tbsp. vinegar
- 1/2 tbsp. dry mustard
- 1 tbsp. lite mayonnaise
- Pepper to taste
- pinch of paprika

Directions:

1. First, place the eggs in a small saucepan with water (it should cover the eggs) and let them cook for 8 minutes from the time they come to a boil.

2. Once the eggs are ready, separate the yolk from the whites and set the whites aside.

3. At this point, mash the yolk with a fork and add to the onion, vinegar, dry

mustard, mayonnaise, and pepper.

4. With the mixture obtained, fill the egg whites previously set aside and sprinkle with paprika.

Calories: 160.32 kcal
Total Fat: 13.67 g
Potassium: 89.18 mg
Sodium: 117.72 mg
Phosphorus: 113.13 mg
Protein: 7.68 g
Total Carbohydrate: 1.38 g
Sugars: 0.89 g
Dietary Fiber: 2.4 g

23. Cream Cheese Omelet

Preparation Time: 10 minutes

Cooking Time: 25 minutes

Servings: 8

Ingredients:

- 1 tsp. butter
- 1/2 tsp. canola oil
- 8 eggs, beaten
- 6 oz. cream cheese
- 1/2 tsp. salt
- 3 tbsp. sour cream
- 1/4 tsp. sage
- 1/4 tsp. dried oregano
- 1 tsp. chives, chopped

Directions:

1. First, take a fairly large skillet and pour in the butter along with the oil and let it heat over medium-low heat until you have a smooth liquid.

2. Meanwhile, in a bowl, combine the salt, sour cream, sage, dried oregano, and chives. Then, add the eggs and mix well with the help of a fork so as to obtain a uniform mixture.

3. At this point, pour the mixture into the pan, sprinkle with the cream cheese and cook for about 20 minutes on low heat.

4. Once this time has elapsed, cut the omelet into slices and serve.

Nutrition Facts Per Serving:

Calories: 148 kcal
Fat: 13.7 g
Fiber: 0 g
Carbs: 0 g
Protein: 12.2 g
Total Carbohydrate: 42 g
Dietary Fiber: 2.4 g

24. Breakfast Potato Latkes with Spinach

Preparation Time: 10 minutes
Cooking Time: 6 minutes
Servings: 4

Ingredients:

- 2 potatoes, peeled
- 1/2 onion, diced
- 1/2 cup spinach, chopped
- 2 eggs, beaten
- 1/2 tsp. salt
- 1/2 tsp. ground black pepper
- 1 tsp. olive oil

Directions:

1. Mash the potatoes using a fork or potato masher and combine with the chopped spinach, diced onion, salt, and ground pepper.
2. Beat the eggs and add them to the potato mixture and stir to make everything smooth.
3. At this point, in a frying pan, pour the oil and heat it well.
4. In the meantime, create the latkes using two spoons and, once the oil is hot, pour them into the pan and cook 3 minutes per side, or until golden brown.
5. Then transfer them to a plate lined with paper towels and enjoy piping hot

Nutrition Facts Per Serving:

Calories: 322 kcal
Fat: 3.5 g

Fiber: 3 g

Protein: 4.9 g

Total Carbohydrates: 25.1 g

Dietary Fiber: 5.2 g

Sodium: 330 mg

Potassium: 520 mg

Phosphorus: 110 mg

25. Healthy, Easy Turnip Puree

Preparation Time: 15 minutes

Cooking Time: 15 minutes

Servings: 4

Ingredients:

- 1 1/2 lbs. turnips, peeled and chopped
- 1 tsp. dill
- 3 turkey bacon slices, cooked and chopped
- 2 tbsp. fresh chives, chopped

Directions:

1. First, get a medium-sized pot and let the water boil. As soon as the water comes to a boil, pour in the well-washed turnips and cook for 15 minutes.

2. After this time, drain the turnips well and place them in a food processor along with the dill.

3. At this point, operate the food processor and blend well until a smooth, homogeneous puree is obtained.

4. Take a glass or ceramic bowl and pour in the puree along with the bacon and chives.

5. Serve.

Nutrition Facts Per Serving:

Calories: 127

Fat: 6 g

Carbohydrates: 11.6 g

Sugar: 7 g

Protein: 5.7 g

Cholesterol: 10 mg

Protein: 5.7 g

Sodium: 380 mg

Potassium: 330 mg

Phosphorus: 46 mg

26. Green Lettuce Bacon Breakfast Bake

Preparation Time: 15 minutes

Cooking Time: 45 minutes

Servings: 6

Ingredients:

- 5 eggs
- 3 cups baby green lettuce, chopped
- 1 tbsp. olive oil
- 8 bacon slices, cooked and chopped
- 2 Red bell peppers, sliced
- 2 tbsp. chives, chopped
- Pepper
- Salt

Directions:

1. First, take a medium-sized baking dish and spray it with cooking spray and set aside; then preheat the oven to 350 F.
2. In a relatively large skillet, pour the oil and add the green lettuce, which should cook until wilted.
3. At this point, take a bowl and add the eggs, salt, and wilted green lettuce. Mix well.
4. Take the baking dish that we had previously set aside and pour the mixture together with the bacon, red peppers, and chives.
5. Let bake for 45 minutes and then serve.

Nutrition Facts Per Serving:

Calories: 273 kcal

Fat: 20.4 g

Carbohydrates: 3.1 g

Sugar: 1.7 g

Protein: 17 g

Cholesterol: 301 mg

Sodium: 720 mg

Potassium: 225 mg

Phosphorus: 161 mg

27. Healthy Green Lettuce Tomato Muffins

Preparation Time: 10 minutes

Cooking Time: 20 minutes

Servings: 12

Ingredients:

- 12 eggs
- 1/2 tsp. Italian seasoning
- 1 cup Red bell peppers, chopped
- 4 tbsp. water
- 1 cup fresh green lettuce, chopped
- ½ tsp pepper
- 1 tsp salt

Directions:

1. First, preheat the oven to 350 F and prepare a muffin tray by spraying the cooking spray.
2. Set the tray aside and move on to the actual preparation.
3. Next, take a mixing bowl and combine the eggs with water, Italian seasoning, pepper, and salt. Mix well, and then add the green lettuce and red peppers.
4. Take the muffin tray again and pour the mixture on top and bake for 20 minutes.
5. Serve.

Nutrition Facts Per Serving:

Calories: 67 kcal

Fat: 4.5 g

Carbohydrates: 1 g

Sugars: 0.8 g

Protein: 5.7 g

Cholesterol: 164 mg

Sodium: 257 mg

Potassium: 94 mg

Phosphorus: 91.5 mg

28. Chicken Egg Breakfast Muffin

Preparation Time: 10 minutes

Cooking Time: 15 minutes

Servings: 12

Ingredients:

- 5 eggs
- 1 cup cooked chicken, chopped
- 3 tbsp. green onions, chopped
- ¼ tsp. garlic powder
- Pepper
- ½ Salt

Directions:

1. Start by getting a muffin tray and spraying cooking spray on it. Also, preheat the oven to 400 F.
2. Now, take a large bowl and combine the eggs with pepper, salt, and garlic powder and mix well.
3. Then add the rest of the ingredients, continuing to mix.
4. When the compote is ready, pour it into the muffin tray and bake for 15 minutes.
5. Serve.

Nutrition Facts Per Serving:

Calories: 571 kcal

Fat: 8 g

Carbohydrates: 0.4 g

Sugar: 0.3 g

Protein: 6.5 g

Cholesterol: 145 mg

Sodium: 91 mg

Potassium: 76.45 mg

Phosphorus: 88.86 mg

29. Breakfast Egg Salad

Preparation Time: 10 minutes

Cooking Time: 8 minutes

Servings: 6

Ingredients:

- 6 large eggs
- 1 tbsp. fresh dill, chopped
- 4 tbsp. lite mayonnaise
- Pepper

- Salt

1. Start by preparing the boiled eggs.
2. Pour eggs into a pot with water and bring to a boil. Cook the eggs for 8 minutes when the water is boiling again.
3. Then, take a large bowl and combine all the ingredients. Stir well to even out all the flavors.
4. Serve.

Nutrition Facts Per Serving:

Calories: 140 kcal
Fat: 10 g
Carbohydrates: 4 g
Sugars: 1 g
Protein: 8 g
Cholesterol: 245 mg
Sodium: 474 mg
Phosphorus: 78 mg
Potassium: 64 mg

30. Healthy Vegetable Tofu Scramble

Preparation Time: 10 minutes
Cooking Time: 7 minutes
Servings: 2

Ingredients:

- 1/2 block firm tofu, crumbled
- 1/4 tsp. ground cumin
- 1 tbsp. turmeric
- 1 cup green lettuce
- 1/4 cup zucchini, chopped
- 1 tbsp. olive oil
- 1 tomato, chopped
- 1 tbsp. chives, chopped
- 1 tbsp. coriander, chopped
- Pepper
- 0.5-1 tsp salt

Directions:

1. Take a frying pan and pour over the oil. Let it heat for a few seconds over medium heat.

2. At this point, add the tomato, zucchini, and green lettuce. Let it fry for about 2 minutes.
3. After this time has elapsed, add the tofu, cumin, turmeric, salt, and pepper. Allow sautéing for another 5 minutes.
4. Season with chives and cilantro and serve.

Nutrition Facts Per Serving:

Calories: 115 kcal
Total Fat: 8.39 g
Carbs: 6.78 g
Sugars: 2.39 g
Protein: 3.72 g
Sodium: 18.04 mg
Potassium: 313 mg
Phosphorus: 41 mg

31. Cheese Coconut Pancake

Preparation Time: 10 minutes
Cooking Time: 8 minutes
Servings: 1

Ingredients:

- 2 eggs
- 1 packet stevia
- 1/2 tsp. cinnamon
- 2 oz. cream cheese
- 1 tbsp. coconut flour
- 1/2 tsp. vanilla

Directions:

1. First, take a bowl and combine all ingredients, whisking to make a smooth mixture. Help yourself with an immersion blender or whisk (it will take longer).
2. Then heat a skillet over medium-high heat, making sure to spray cooking spray on top.
3. At this point, pour the mixture into the hot skillet and cook until the

first bubbles appear. At that point, flip the pancake over and cook on the other side until it is slightly brown.

4. Remove from the skillet and serve piping hot.

Nutrition Facts Per Serving:

Calories: 181.91 kcal

Fat: 14.46 g

Carbohydrates: 5.54 g

Sugars: 1.88 g

Protein: 7.8 g

Cholesterol: 389 m

Potassium: 102 mg

Phosphorus: 117 mg

Sodium: 154.15 mg

32. Cheesy Scrambled Eggs with Fresh Herbs

Preparation Time: 10 minutes

Cooking Time: 5 minutes

Servings: 4

Ingredients:

- Eggs 3
- Egg whites 2
- Cream cheese 1/2 cup
- Unsweetened rice milk 1/4 cup
- Chopped scallion 1 Tbsp. green part only
- Chopped fresh tarragon 1 Tbsp.
- Unsalted butter 2 tsp.
- Ground black pepper to taste

Directions:

1. Take a bowl and combine the whole eggs and the egg whites, cream cheese, rice milk, scallion, and tarragon. Mix until smooth and homogeneous.

2. At this point, place the butter in a skillet and let it melt over low heat.

3. Once the butter is melted, add the egg mixture and cook for 5 minutes, taking care to stir, until the eggs are cooked, and everything is creamy.

4. Finish with pepper and serve.

Nutrition Facts Per Serving:

Calories: 221 kcal
Fat: 19 g
Carbs: 3 g
Phosphorus: 119 mg
Potassium: 140 mg
Sodium: 193 mg
Protein: 8 g

33. Coconut Breakfast Smoothie

Preparation Time: 5 minutes
Cooking Time: 0 minutes
Servings: 1

Ingredients:

- 1/4 cup whey protein powder
- 1/2 cup coconut milk
- 5 drops liquid stevia
- 1 tbsp. coconut oil
- 1 tsp. vanilla
- 2 tbsp. coconut butter
- 1/4 cup water
- 1/2 cup ice

Directions:

1. Attach all ingredients into the blender and blend until smooth.
2. Serve and enjoy.

Nutrition Facts Per Serving:

Calories: 560 kcal
Fat: 45 g
Carbohydrates: 12 g
Sugar: 4 g
Protein: 25 g
Cholesterol: 60 mg
Sodium: 41.5 mg
Potassium: 153 mg
Phosphorus: 91.5 mg

34. Turkey and Green Lettuce Scramble on Melba Toast

Preparation Time: 2 minutes

Cooking Time: 14 minutes

Servings: 2

Ingredients:

- 1 tsp Extra virgin olive oil
- Raw green lettuce 1 cup
- Garlic 1/2 clove, minced
- Nutmeg 1 tsp. grated
- Cooked and diced turkey breast 1 cup
- Melba toast 2 slices
- Balsamic vinegar 1 tsp.

Directions:

1. Heat the oil in a skillet over medium-high heat.
2. As soon as the oil is hot, add the already cooked and diced turkey and cook for 6-8 minutes.
3. At this point, add the garlic, green lettuce, and nutmeg and cook for another 6 minutes.
4. Place the Melba Toast on a plate and add the turkey and green lettuce as soon as they are ready.
5. Drizzle with balsamic vinegar and serve.

Nutrition Facts Per Serving:

Calories: 301 kcal

Fat: 19 g

Carb: 12 g

Phosphorus: 215 mg

Potassium: 269 mg

Sodium: 360 mg

Protein: 19 g

35. Vegetable Healthy Omelet

Preparation Time: 15 minutes

Cooking Time: 10 minutes

Servings: 3

Ingredients:

- Egg whites 4
- Egg 1

- Chopped fresh parsley 2 Tbsps.
- Water 2 Tbsps.
- Olive oil spray
- Chopped and boiled red bell pepper 1/2 cup
- Chopped scallion 1/4 cup, both green and white parts
- Ground black pepper

Directions:

1. First, take a bowl and combine the egg along with the egg whites and water. Whisk the mixture until all the ingredients are well blended.
2. Separately, heat a skillet over medium heat with cooking spray.
3. As soon as the skillet is hot, pour in the peppers and shallots, and sauté for 3 minutes until they have reached a morbid consistency.
4. At this point, pour the egg mixture into the skillet and cook until they have reached a thick consistency.
5. Season with black pepper and serve.

Nutrition Facts Per Serving:

Calories: 112.82 kcal
Fat: 6.36 g
Carbs: 4.22 g
Sugars: 2.37 g
Phosphorus: 68.8 mg
Potassium: 250 mg
Sodium: 132.89 mg
Protein: 9.81 g

36. Mexican Style Burritos

Preparation Time: 5 minutes

Cooking Time: 15 minutes

Servings: 2

Ingredients:

- Olive oil 1 Tbsp.
- 2 Corn tortillas
- Red onion 1/4 cup, chopped
- Red bell peppers 1/4 cup, chopped

- Red chili 1/2, deseeded and chopped
- Eggs 2
- Juice of 1 lime
- Cilantro 1 Tbsp. chopped

Directions:

1. Heat a grill over medium heat and arrange the tortillas. Let them heat for 1 to 2 minutes on each side until lightly toasted.
2. Meanwhile, take a skillet and sauté the onion along with the red chili and afterward add the peppers and cook for 5 0 6 minutes, until soft.
3. Also, add the eggs to the skillet and cook for another 10 minutes until the eggs are fully cooked.
4. Divide the egg and vegetable mixture between the two tortillas, sprinkle with cilantro and lime juice and serve.

Nutrition Facts Per Serving:

Calories: 202 kcal

Fat: 13 g
Carb: 19 g
Phosphorus: 184 mg
Potassium: 233 mg
Sodium: 77 mg
Protein: 9 g

37. Healthy Bulgur, Couscous and Buckwheat Cereal

Preparation Time: 10 minutes

Cooking Time: 25 minutes

Servings: 4

Ingredients:

- Water 2 1/4 cups
- Vanilla rice milk 1 1/4 cups
- Uncooked bulgur 6 Tbsps.
- Uncooked whole buckwheat 2 Tbsps.
- Sliced apple 1 cup
- Plain uncooked couscous 6 Tbsps.
- Ground cinnamon 1/2 tsp.

Directions:

1. Fill a saucepan with the water and milk and bring to a boil over medium heat. Once it comes to a boil, add the bulgur, apple, buckwheat, and couscous.
2. At this point, lower the heat and simmer for 20-25 minutes, taking care to stir occasionally.
3. As soon as bulgur is tender and grains are cooked, remove the saucepan from heat, add cinnamon and stir again. Finally, let everything rest with the lid on.
4. Before serving, be sure to stem the grains with a fork.

Nutrition Facts Per Serving:

Calories: 347.54 kcal
Fat: 2.45 g
Carbs: 74.22 g
Sugars: 13.94 g
Phosphorus: 260 mg

Potassium: 308 mg
Sodium: 71.75 mg
Protein: 9.35 g

38.   Sweet Pancakes

Preparation Time: 10 minutes

Cooking Time: 4 minutes

Servings: 5

Ingredients:

- 1 cup All-purpose flour
- 1 Tbsp Granulated sugar
- 2 Tsps. Baking powder.
- 2 Egg whites
- 1 cup Unsweetened Almond milk
- 2 Tbsps. Olive oil
- 1 Tbsp Maple extract

Directions:

1. Take two bowls and mix the flour, sugar, and baking powder in one bowl; in another, the egg whites, milk, oil, and maple extract.
2. At this point, take the bowl with the flour mixture and make a well

in the center and pour the egg mixture into it, making sure to stir, so you get a smooth, even batter.

3. Next, take a non-stick skillet and heat it on the stove. Then, pour in 1/5 of the batter, and cook the first pancake for 2 minutes on each side.

4. Repeat the same process with the remaining batter to make the other pancakes.

5. Serve.

Nutrition Facts Per Serving:

Calories: 445.04 kcal
Fat: 16.27 g
Carbs: 64.08 g
Sugars: 14.8 g
Phosphorus: 183.6 mg
Potassium: 180.2 mg
Sodium: 619.89 mg
Protein: 10.17 g

39. Breakfast Smoothie

Preparation Time: 15 minutes

Cooking Time: 0 minutes

Servings: 2

Ingredients:

- Frozen blueberries 1/2 cup
- Pineapple chunks 1/2 cup
- English cucumber 1/2 cup
- Apple 1/2
- Water 1/2 cup

Directions:

1. Put the pineapple, blueberries, cucumber, apple, and water in a blender and blend until thick and smooth.

2. Pour into 2 glasses and serve.

Nutrition Facts Per Serving:

Calories: 87 kcal
Fat: 0.4 g
Carbs: 22 g

Phosphorus: 28 mg
Potassium: 192 mg
Sodium: 3 mg
Protein: 0.7 g

40. Buckwheat and Grapefruit Porridge

Preparation Time: 5 minutes

Cooking Time: 20 minutes

Servings: 2

Ingredients:

- Buckwheat 1/2 cup
- Water 2 cups
- Almond milk 1 1/2 cups
- Grapefruit –1/4, chopped
- Honey 1 Tbsp.

Directions:

1. Take a saucepan and put the water to boil over medium heat. Once the water is boiling, add the buckwheat and cover the pot with the lid.
2. Lower the heat and simmer for 7-10 minutes, making sure the water doesn't dry out.
3. As soon as most of the water is absorbed, turn off the stove and set it aside for 5 minutes.
4. Drain the excess water from the saucepan and add the almond milk, stirring and heating for 5 minutes.
5. Add the honey and grapefruit.
6. Serve.

Nutrition Facts per Serving:

Calories: 231 kcal
Fat: 4 g
Carbs: 43 g
Phosphorus: 165 mg
Potassium: 370 mg
Sodium: 135 mg

41. Egg and Veggie Muffins

Preparation Time: 15 minutes

Cooking Time: 20 minutes

Servings: 4

Ingredients:

- 1 puff cooking oil spray
- Eggs 4
- Unsweetened rice milk 2 Tbsp.
- Sweet onion 1/2, chopped
- Red bell pepper 1/2, chopped
- a sprig of parsley
- Pinch red pepper flakes
- Pinch ground black pepper

Directions:

1. First, be sure to preheat the oven to 350F.

2. Next, take four muffin pans and spray with cooking spray. Set aside.

3. In a bowl, combine the milk, eggs, onion, red bell pepper, parsley, red bell pepper flakes, and black pepper and mix well.

4. Pour the egg mixture into the previously prepared muffin pans and bake for about 10-20 minutes until the muffins are puffy and golden brown.

5. Serve.

Nutrition Facts per Serving:

Calories: 184 kcal

Fat: 5 g

Carbs: 3 g

Phosphorus: 110 mg

Potassium: 117 mg

Sodium: 75 mg

Protein: 7 g

Lunch

42. Chicken and Mushroom Stew

Preparation Time: 10 minutes

Cooking Time: 35 minutes

Servings: 4

Ingredients:

- 2 chicken breast halves
- 1 pound mushrooms, sliced (5-6 cups)
- 1 bunch spring onion, chopped
- 4 tablespoons olive oil
- 1 teaspoon thyme
- Salt and pepper as needed

Directions:

1. First, heat the oil in a large deep pan over medium-high heat.
2. After that, add the chicken and cook for 4-5 minutes per side until lightly browned.
3. At this point, add the spring onions and mushrooms and season with salt and pepper, depending on your taste.
4. Next, mix well and then put the lid on and bring to a boil.
5. Lower the heat and simmer for 25 minutes.
6. Serve.

Nutrition Facts Per Serving:

Calories: 850.36 kcal
Fat: 58.04 g
Carbohydrates: 10.79 g
Sugars: 5.54 g
Protein: 72.49 g
Sodium: 214.45 mg
Potassium: 1530.13 mg
Phosphorus: 750 mg

43. Roasted Carrot Soup

Preparation Time: 10 minutes

Cooking Time: 45 minutes

Servings: 4

Ingredients:

- 8 large carrots, washed and peeled

- 6 tablespoons olive oil
- 1-quart broth
- Cayenne pepper to taste
- Salt and pepper to taste

Directions:

1. First, preheat the oven to 425 F.
2. Then, on a baking sheet, add the carrots and drizzle them with olive oil. Bake the carrots and let them cook for 30-45 minutes.
3. After the carrots are cooked, place them in a blender and add the broth. Then, blend and reduce to a puree.
4. Heat the puree in a saucepan and season with salt, pepper, and cayenne.
5. Drizzle with olive oil and serve.

Nutrition Facts per Serving:

Calories: 510.8 kcal
Fat: 43.92 g
Carbohydrates: 29.55 g
Sugars: 14.8 g

Protein: 3.81 g
Sodium: 2239.24 mg
Potassium: 916 mg
Phosphorus: 106 mg

44. Healthy Garlic and Butter-flavored Cod

Preparation Time: 5 minutes

Cooking Time: 20 minutes

Servings: 3

Ingredients:

- 3 Cod fillets, 8 ounces each
- 3/4 pound baby bok choy halved
- 1/3 cup almond butter, thinly sliced
- 1 1/2 tablespoons garlic, minced
- Salt and pepper to taste

Directions:

1. First, preheat the oven to 400 F.
2. Take some aluminum foil and cut out three sheets

80

(large enough to fit the fillet).

3. Lay the cod fillet on each sheet and add the butter and garlic on top.
4. After that, add the bok choy and season with pepper and salt.
5. Fold the aluminum foil over and create pouches to place on a baking sheet. Then, bake for 20 minutes.
6. After these minutes are up, place the bags with the cod on a cooling rack and allow them to cool.
7. Serve.

Nutrition Facts per Serving:

Calories: 554.78 kcal
Fat: 25.53 g
Carbohydrates: 14.72 g
Protein: 72.46 g
Sodium: 897.07 mg
Potassium: 318.49 mg
Phosphorus: 212.52 mg

45. Healthy Tilapia Broccoli Platter

Preparation Time: 4 minutes
Cooking Time: 15 minutes
Servings: 2

Ingredients:

- 6 ounces of tilapia, frozen
- 1 cup of broccoli florets, fresh
- 1 teaspoon of lemon pepper seasoning
- 1 tablespoon of almond butter
- 1 tablespoon of garlic, minced

Directions:

1. First, preheat the oven to 350 F.
2. Then, add fish in foil packets and arrange broccoli around the fish.
3. After that, sprinkle with lemon pepper and close the packets, sealing well.
4. Allow cooking for about 15 minutes.
5. Meanwhile, in a bowl, add the garlic and butter, mix

well and keep the mixture aside.

6. Remove the packets from the oven and transfer them to a serving dish.
7. Place the butter on top of the fish and broccoli, serve and enjoy!

Nutrition Facts per Serving:

Calories: 146.99 kcal
Fat: 5.92 g
Carbohydrates: 2 g
Protein: 19.72 g
Sodium: 305.44 mg
Potassium: 400 mg
Phosphorus: 200 mg

46. Parsley Scallops

Preparation Time: 5 minutes

Cooking Time: 25 minutes

Servings: 4

Ingredients:

- 16 large sea scallops
- 1 1/2 tablespoons olive oil
- Salt and pepper to taste
- 8 tablespoons almond butter
- 2 garlic cloves, minced

Directions:

1. In a skillet, add the oil and heat over medium heat. Meanwhile, Season the scallops with salt and pepper.
2. Once the oil is hot, sauté the scallops for 2 minutes on each side and repeat the same process with all the scallops. Once cooked, remove the scallops from the pan and add the butter to the pan to melt.
3. Add the garlic and cook for 15 minutes.
4. Return the scallops to the pan and stir to coat.
5. Serve and enjoy!

Nutrition Facts per Serving:

Calories: 409 kcal
Fat: 24.91 g
Carbohydrates: 13.36 g
Protein: 34 g

Sodium: 1382.42 mg

Potassium: 600 mg

Phosphorus: 900 mg

47. Blackened Chicken

Preparation Time: 10 minutes

Cooking Time: 10 minutes

Servings: 4

Ingredients:

- 1/2 teaspoon paprika
- 1/8 teaspoon salt
- 1/4 teaspoon cayenne pepper
- 1/4 teaspoon ground cumin
- 1/4 teaspoon dried thyme
- 1/8 teaspoon ground white pepper
- 1/8 teaspoon onion powder
- 2 chicken breasts, boneless and skinless
- 2 tsp. olive oil

Directions:

1. First, grease a baking sheet and preheat the oven to 350 F.
2. Take a cast-iron skillet and heat ½ tsp. of oil for 5 minutes on high heat.
3. Meanwhile, take a small bowl and mix salt, paprika, cumin, white pepper, cayenne, thyme, onion powder.
4. Then, oil the chicken breast on both sides and coat the breast with the spice mix.
5. Transfer the chicken to the hot pan and cook for 1 minute per side.
6. Transfer to the prepared baking sheet and bake for 5 minutes.
7. Serve and enjoy!

Nutrition Facts per Serving:

Calories: 136 kcal

Fat: 5 g

Carbohydrates: 1 g

Protein: 44 g

Potassium: 690 mg

Phosphorus: 430 mg

Sodium: 240 mg

48. Spicy Paprika Lamb Chops

Preparation Time: 10 minutes

Cooking Time: 10 minutes

Servings: 4

Ingredients:

- 0.5 lb. lamb racks, cut into chops
- Salt and pepper to taste
- 3 tablespoons paprika
- 3/4 cup cumin powder
- 1 teaspoon chili powder

Directions:

1. Mix the paprika, cumin, chili, salt, and pepper inside a bowl.
2. Add the lamb chops and allow the spice mixture to adhere to the lamb.
3. Heat a grill to medium temperature and add the lamb chops; cook for 5 minutes.
4. Turn and cook for another 5 minutes.
5. Serve and enjoy!

Nutrition Facts Per Serving:

Calories: 529.25 kcal

Fat: 37.34 g

Carbohydrates: 22.7 g

Protein: 108.72 g

Sodium: 585.4 mg

Potassium: 600 mg

Phosphorus: 400 mg

49. Healthy Mushroom and Olive Sirloin Steak

Preparation Time: 10 minutes

Cooking Time: 14 minutes

Servings: 4

Ingredients:

- 1 pound boneless beef sirloin steak
- 1 large red onion, chopped
- 1 cup mushrooms

- 4 garlic cloves, thinly sliced
- 4 tablespoons olive oil
- 1 cup parsley leaves, finely cut

Directions:

1. Heat 2 tbsp. oil over medium-high heat in a large skillet.
2. Add the beef and cook until both sides are browned; remove the beef from the skillet and discard the fat.
3. At this point, add the rest of the oil to the skillet and heat it.
4. Add the onions and garlic and cook for 2-3 minutes, stirring well.
5. Return the beef to the skillet and lower the heat to medium.
6. Cook for 3-4 minutes with the lid on.
7. Garnish with parsley.
8. Serve and enjoy!

Nutrition Facts Per Serving:

Calories: 754.46 kcal
Fat: 57.82 g
Carbohydrates: 8.09 g
Sugars: 3 g
Protein: 49.58 g
Sodium: 140.58 mg
Potassium: 1168.62 mg
Phosphorus: 512 mg

50. Healthy Parsley and Chicken Breast

Preparation Time: 10 minutes
Cooking Time: 30 minutes
Servings: 4

Ingredients:

- 1 tablespoon dry parsley
- 1 tablespoon dry basil
- 4 chicken breast halves, boneless and skinless
- 1 garlic clove, sliced
- 1/2 teaspoon salt
- 1/2 teaspoon red pepper flakes, crushed

Directions:

1. First, preheat your oven to 350 F and prepare a 9x13-inch baking dish by greasing it with cooking spray.
2. Sprinkle one teaspoon parsley and one teaspoon basil on the baking sheet and arrange the chicken breast halves, spreading the garlic slices on top.
3. Take a small bowl and add one teaspoon parsley, one teaspoon basil, salt, red pepper, and mix well. Pour mixture over chicken breast.
4. Bake for 30 minutes.
5. Serve and enjoy!

Nutrition Facts Per Serving:

Calories: 560.55 kcal
Fat: 8 g
Carbohydrates: 0.4 g
Sugars: 0.7 g
Protein: 80.38 g
Sodium: 675.6 mg
Potassium: 734.35 mg

Phosphorus: 430 mg

51. Simple Mustard Chicken

Preparation Time: 10 minutes
Cooking Time: 35 minutes
Servings: 4

Ingredients:

- 3 chicken breasts
- 1/2 cup chicken broth
- 3-4 tablespoons mustard
- 2 tablespoons olive oil
- 1 teaspoon paprika
- 1 teaspoon chili powder
- 1 teaspoon garlic powder

Directions:

1. Combine the mustard, olive oil, paprika, chicken broth, garlic powder, chili powder in a small bowl to create an emulsion.
2. At this point, pour the emulsion over the chicken breasts and let marinate for 30 minutes.

3. Line a large baking sheet with parchment paper and arrange the chicken.
4. Bake for 35 minutes at 375 F
5. Serve and enjoy!

Nutrition Facts Per Serving:

Calories: 750 kcal
Fat: 80 g
Carbohydrates: 2 g
Protein: 130 g
Potassium: 1410.51 mg
Phosphorus: 1106.42 mg

52. Healthy Golden Eggplant Fries

Preparation Time: 10 minutes
Cooking Time: 15 minutes
Servings: 8

Ingredients:

- 2 eggs
- 2 cups almond flour
- Sunflower seeds and pepper
- 2 tablespoons coconut oil, spray
- 2 eggplants, peeled and cut thinly

Directions:

1. First, preheat the oven to 400 degrees F.
2. Next, mix the almond flour with the sunflower seeds and black pepper in a bowl.
3. Separately, beat the eggs in another bowl until frothy.
4. Dip the eggplant pieces into the eggs and toss them in the flour mixture.
5. Next, dip the eggplant again, first in the egg and then in the flour.
6. Take a baking sheet, grease it with coconut oil on top and arrange the eggplants.
7. Bake for about 15 minutes.
8. Serve.

Nutrition Facts Per Serving:

Calories: 855.72 kcal
Total Fat: 69.01 g

Carbs: 42.53 g

Sugars: 16.86 g

Protein: 30.63 g

Sodium: 69.88 mg

Potassium: 1543.09 mg

Phosphorus: 200.82 mg

53. Very Wild Mushroom Pilaf

Note: To make this recipe, a Slow Cooker is needed; alternatively, a Dutch oven or any heavy-duty pot with a good lid will work.

Preparation Time: 10 minutes

Cooking Time: 3 hours

Servings: 4

Ingredients:

- 1 cup wild rice
- 2 garlic cloves, minced
- 6 green onions, chopped
- 2 tablespoons olive oil
- 1/2 pound baby Bella mushrooms
- 2 cups water

Directions using Slow Cooker:

1. Add rice, garlic, onion, oil, mushrooms and water to your Slow Cooker.
2. Stir well until mixed.
3. Set the lid and cook on LOW for 3 hours.
4. Stir pilaf and divide between serving platters.
5. Enjoy!

Directions using other pots:

1. Sauté the oil in your pot along with the garlic and onion. Once the onion is nicely browned, add the mushrooms and cook for a few minutes. At that point, add the rice and let it blanch.
2. In the meantime, have the water heated in another small pot.
3. Once the rice has taken on some color, gradually pour the hot water into the pot and continue stirring until the rice is

fully cooked. This will take about 30 minutes.

4. Serve.

Nutrition Facts Per Serving:

Calories: 210 kcal
Fat: 7 g
Carbohydrates: 16 g
Protein: 4 g
Phosphorus: 110 mg
Potassium: 117 mg
Sodium: 75 mg

54.   Sporty Baby Carrots

Preparation Time: 5 minutes

Cooking Time: 5 minutes

Servings: 4

Ingredients:

- 1-pound baby carrots
- 1 cup water
- 1 tablespoon clarified ghee
- 1 tablespoon chopped up fresh mint leaves
- Sea flavored vinegar as needed

Directions:

1. Set a steamer rack on top of your pot and add the carrots.
2. Add water.
3. Lock the lid and cook at HIGH pressure for 2 minutes. Do a quick release.
4. Pass the carrots through a strainer and drain them.
5. Wipe the insert clean.
6. Set the insert to the pot and set the pot to Sauté mode.
7. Add clarified butter and allow it to melt.
8. Add mint and sauté for 30 seconds.
9. Add carrots to the insert and sauté well.
10. Remove them and sprinkle a bit of flavored vinegar on top.
11. Enjoy!

Nutrition Facts Per Serving:

Calories: 131 kcal
Fat: 10 g
Carbohydrates: 11 g

Protein: 1 g
Sodium: 85 mg
Phosphorus: 130 mg
Potassium: 147 mg

55. Saucy Garlic Greens

Preparation Time: 5 minutes

Cooking Time: 20 minutes

Servings: 4

Ingredients:

- 1/2 cup cashews
- 1/4 cup water
- 1 tablespoon lemon juice
- 1 teaspoon coconut aminos
- 1 clove peeled whole clove
- 1/8 teaspoon of flavored vinegar
- 1 bunch of leafy greens
- lite Sauce

Directions:

1. Drain and discard the soaking water from your cashews and add them to a blender to make the sauce.
2. Add fresh water, lemon juice, flavored vinegar, coconut aminos, and garlic.
3. Blend to obtain a smooth cream and transfer to a bowl.
4. Add 1/2 cup of water to the pot and place a steamer basket on it.
5. Add the greens to the basket.
6. Lock the lid and steam for 1 minute. Quick release the pressure.
7. Transfer the steamed greens to a strainer and extract excess water.
8. Place the greens into a mixing bowl.
9. Add lemon, garlic, sauce and toss.
10. Serve.

Nutrition Facts Per Serving:

Calories: 196.65 kcal
Fat: 15.88 g
Carbohydrates: 11.2 g

90

Sugars: 1.72 g

Protein: 5.25 g

Phosphorus: 167.87 mg

Potassium: 193.57 mg

Sodium: 5.48 mg

56. Pasta with Creamy Broccoli Sauce

Preparation Time: 15 minutes

Cooking Time: 40 minutes

Servings: 2

Ingredients:

- 1 tbsp. olive oil
- 0.25 lb. broccoli florets
- 1 1/2 garlic cloves, halved
- 1/2 cup low-sodium vegetable broth
- 1/4 cup whole-wheat spaghetti pasta
- 2 tbsp cream cheese
- 1/2 tsp. dried basil leaves

Directions:

1. Take a pot and set water to a boil to cook your pasta.

2. Meanwhile, put olive oil in a large skillet and sauté the broccoli with the garlic for 3 minutes.

3. Then, add the broth to the skillet and bring it to a simmer. Reduce the heat to low, partially cover the skillet, and simmer until the broccoli is tender; it will take about 5–6 minutes.

4. Cook the pasta according to package directions or for 12 minutes. Drain when al dente, reserving 1 cup pasta water.

5. When the broccoli is tender, add the cream cheese, basil, and purée using an immersion blender.

6. Put the mixture into a food processor, about half at a time, and purée until smooth; then, transfer the sauce back into the skillet.

7. Add the cooked pasta to the broccoli sauce. Toss, adding enough pasta water until the sauce coats

the pasta thoroughly.
Serve

Nutrition Facts Per Serving:

Calories: 410 kcal

Fats: 26 g

Carbs: 36 g

Protein: 11 g

Sodium: 260 mg

Potassium: 900 mg

Phosphorus: 223 mg

57. Delicious Vegetarian Lasagna

Preparation time: 10 minutes

Cooking time: 1 ¼ hour

Servings: 4

Ingredients:

- 1 teaspoon basil
- 1 tablespoon olive oil
- 1/2 sliced red pepper
- 2 lasagna sheets
- 1/2 diced red onion
- 1/4 teaspoon black pepper
- 1 cup rice milk
- 1 minced garlic clove
- 1 cup sliced eggplant
- 1/2 sliced zucchini
- 1/2 pack soft tofu
- 1 teaspoon oregano

Directions:

1. Preheat the oven to 325f. or if gas, mark 3.
2. Slice zucchini, eggplant and pepper into vertical strips.
3. Add the rice milk and tofu to a food processor and blitz until smooth. Set aside.
4. Warm up the oil and add the onions and garlic for 3-4 minutes or until soft.
5. Sprinkle in the herbs (oregano) and pepper and allow to stir through for 5-6 minutes until hot.
6. Into a lasagna or suitable oven dish, layer 1 lasagna sheet, then 1/3 the eggplant, followed by 1/3 zucchini, then 1/3 pepper

92

before pouring over 1/3 of tofu white sauce.

7. Repeat for the next 2 layers, finishing with the white sauce.

8. Add to the oven for 40-50 minutes or until the veg is soft and can easily be sliced into servings.

Nutrition Facts Per Serving:

Calories: 235 kcal
Protein: 5 g
Carbs: 10 g
Fat: 9 g
Sodium: 35 mg
Potassium: 129 mg
Phosphorus: 66 mg

58. Creamy Pesto Pasta

Preparation time: 10 minutes

Cooking time: 20 minutes

Servings: 4

Ingredients:

- 4 ounces linguine noodles
- 2 cups packed basil leaves
- 2 cups packed arugula leaves
- 1/3 cup walnut pieces
- 3 garlic cloves
- 3 tbsp. extra-virgin olive oil
- Freshly ground black pepper

Directions:

1. Set a medium stock pot halfway with water, and bring to a boil. Cook the noodles al dente, for about 10-12 minutes and drain.

2. In a food processor, add the basil, arugula, walnuts, and garlic. Process until coarsely ground. With the food processor running, slowly add the olive oil, and continue to mix until creamy. Season with pepper.

3. Merge the noodles with the pesto and serve.

Nutrition Facts Per Serving:

Calories: 394 kcal

93

Total Fat: 21 g

Saturated Fat: 3 g

Cholesterol: 0 mg

Carbohydrates: 0 g

Fiber: 3 g

Protein: 10 g

Phosphorus: 54 mg

Potassium: 148 mg

Sodium: 4 mg

59. Garden Salad

Preparation Time: 5 minutes

Cooking Time: 20 minutes

Servings: 4

Ingredients:

- 5 oz. raw peanuts in shell
- 1 bay leaf
- 1 medium-sized chopped up Red bell peppers
- 5 tablespoons, 1 teaspoon diced up green pepper
- 5 tablespoons, 1 teaspoon diced up sweet onion
- 2 tablespoons, 2 teaspoons finely diced hot pepper
- 2 tablespoons, 2 teaspoons diced up celery
- 1 tablespoon, 1 teaspoon olive oil
- 0.5 teaspoon flavored vinegar
- 1/4 teaspoon freshly ground black pepper

Directions:

1. Boil your peanuts for 1 minute and rinse them.
2. Their skin will be soft, so discard the skin.
3. Attach 2 cups of water to the Instant Pot.
4. Add bay leaf and peanuts.
5. Lock the lid and cook on HIGH pressure for 20 minutes. Drain the water.
6. Take a large bowl and add the peanuts, diced up vegetables.
7. Whisk in olive oil, lemon juice, pepper in another bowl.
8. Stream the mixture over the salad and mix!
9. Enjoy!

Nutrition Facts Per Serving:

Calories: 240 kcal

Fat: 4 g

Carbohydrates: 24 g

Protein: 5 g

Phosphorus: 110 mg

Potassium: 117 mg

Sodium: 75 mg

60. Zucchini Pasta

Preparation Time: 15 minutes

Cooking Time: 30 Minutes

Servings: 4

Ingredients:

- 3 Tablespoons of olive oil
- 2 Cloves garlic, minced
- 3 Zucchini, large and diced
- Sea salt and black pepper to taste
- 1/2 Cup of 2% milk
- 1/4 Teaspoon of nutmeg
- 1 Tablespoon of lemon juice, fresh
- 1/2 Cup of cheddar, grated
- 8 Ounces uncooked farfalle pasta

Directions:

1. Get out a skillet and place it over medium heat, and then heat up the oil. Attach in your garlic and cook for a minute. Stir often so that it doesn't burn. Add in your salt, pepper, and zucchini. Stir well, and cook covered for fifteen minutes. During this time, you'll want to stir the mixture twice.

2. Get out a microwave-safe bowl, and heat the milk for thirty seconds. Stir in your nutmeg, and then pour it into the skillet. Cook uncovered for five minutes. Stir occasionally to keep from burning.

3. Get out a stockpot and cook your pasta per package instructions. Drain the pasta, and then save two tablespoons of pasta water.

4. Stir everything together, and add in the cheese, and

lemon juice and pasta water.

Calories: 813.76 kcal
Total Fat: 34.79 g
Carbs: 99.71 g
Sugars: 13.74 g
Protein: 27.15 g
Sodium: 577.9 mg
Potassium: 1000 mg
Phosphorus: 500 mg

61. Spicy Cabbage Dish (Healthy)

Note: To make this recipe, a Slow Cooker is needed; alternatively, a Dutch oven or any heavy-duty pot with a good lid will work.

Preparation Time: 10 minutes

Cooking Time: 4 hours

Servings: 4

Ingredients:

- 2 yellow onions, chopped
- 10 cups red cabbage, shredded
- 1 cup plums, pitted and chopped
- 1 teaspoon cinnamon powder
- 1 garlic clove, minced
- 1 teaspoon cumin seeds
- 1/4 teaspoon cloves, ground
- 2 tablespoons red wine vinegar
- 1 teaspoon coriander seeds
- 1/2 cup water

Directions:

1. Combine cabbage, onion, plums, garlic, cumin, cinnamon, cloves, vinegar, coriander, and water to your Slow Cooker.
2. Stir well.
3. Place lid and cook on LOW for 4 hours.
4. Divide between serving platters.
5. Serve.

Calories: 219.48 kcal

Fat: 1.38 g

Carbohydrates: 51.05 g

Protein: 3 g

Phosphorus: 183 mg

Potassium: 1350 mg

Sodium: 113.37 mg

62. Extreme Balsamic Chicken (Healthy)

Preparation Time: 10 minutes

Cooking Time: 25 minutes

Servings: 2

Ingredients:

- 3 boneless chicken breasts, skinless
- 2 tbsp. almond flour
- 1/3 cup low-fat chicken broth
- 1 teaspoon arrowroot
- 1/4 cup low sugar raspberry preserve
- 1 tablespoon balsamic vinegar

Directions:

1. Slice chicken breast into bite-sized pieces and season them with seeds.
2. Dredge the chicken pieces in flour and shake off any excess.
3. Set a non-stick skillet and place it over medium heat.
4. Add chicken to the skillet and cook for 10 minutes, making sure to turn them halfway through.
5. Remove chicken and transfer to a platter.
6. Add arrowroot, broth, raspberry preserve to the skillet and stir.
7. Stir in balsamic vinegar and reduce heat to low; stir-cook for a few minutes.
8. Transfer the chicken back to the sauce and cook for 10 minutes more.
9. Serve.

Nutrition Facts Per Serving:

Calories: 546 kcal

Fat: 35 g

Carbohydrates: 11 g

Protein: 44 g

Phosphorus: 120 mg

Potassium: 117 mg

Sodium: 85 mg

63. Enjoyable Green Lettuce and Bean Medley

Note: To make this recipe, a Slow Cooker is needed; alternatively, a Dutch oven or any heavy duty pot with a good lid will work.

Preparation Time: 10 minutes

Cooking Time: 4 hours

Servings: 2

Ingredients:

- 3 carrots, sliced
- 1 cup great northern beans, dried
- 1 garlic clove, minced
- 1/2 yellow onion, chopped
- Pepper to taste
- 1/4 teaspoon oregano, dried
- 2.5 ounces baby green lettuce
- 2 1/2 cups low sodium veggie stock
- 1 teaspoon lemon peel, grated
- 1 1/2 tablespoon lemon juice

Directions:

1. Combine beans, onion, carrots, garlic, oregano, and stock to your Slow Cooker.
2. Stir well.
3. Set the lid and cook on HIGH for 4 hours.
4. Add green lettuce, lemon juice, and lemon peel.
5. Stir and let it sit for 8 minutes.
6. Divide between serving platters and serve!

Nutrition Facts Per Serving:

Calories: 570.63 kcal

Fat: 2.17 g

Carbohydrates: 110.17 g

Protein: 33.13 g

Phosphorus: 700 mg

Potassium: 1500 mg
Sodium: 145.82 mg

64. Cauliflower and Dill Mash (Healthy, Low Caloric)

Note: To make this recipe, a Slow Cooker is needed; alternatively, a Dutch oven or any heavy-duty pot with a good lid will work.

Preparation Time: 10 minutes
Cooking Time: 5 hours
Servings: 3

Ingredients:

- 1/2 cauliflower head, florets separated
- 2 tbsp. + 2 tsp. cup dill, chopped
- 3 garlic cloves
- 1 tablespoon olive oil
- Pinch of black pepper

Directions:

1. Add cauliflower to Slow Cooker.
2. Add dill, garlic and water to cover them.
3. Place the lid and cook on HIGH for 5 hours.
4. Drain the flowers.
5. Season with pepper and add oil, mash using potato masher.
6. Whisk and serve.

Nutrition Facts Per Serving:

Calories: 42.74 kcal
Fat: 3.03 g
Carbohydrates: 3.55 g
Protein: 1.26 g
Phosphorus: 28.84 mg
Potassium: 185.43 mg
Sodium: 18.19 mg

65. Peas Soup

Preparation Time: 10 minutes
Cooking Time: 10 minutes
Servings: 2

Ingredients:

- 1/2 white onion, chopped
- 1/2 tsp. olive oil
- 1/2 quart veggie stock

- 1 egg
- 1 1/2 tablespoons lemon juice
- 1 cup peas
- 1 tablespoons parmesan, grated
- Salt and black pepper to the taste

Directions:

1. Take a pot and heat 1 tsp. oil over medium-high heat
2. Then, add the onion and sauté for 4 minutes.
3. Attach the rest of the ingredients except the eggs, bring to a simmer, and cook for 4 minutes more.
4. Add whisked eggs, stir the soup, cook for 2 minutes more, divide into bowls and serve.

Nutrition Facts Per Serving:

Calories: 264 kcal
Fat: 7.2 g
Fiber: 3.4 g
Carbs: 33 g
Protein: 17 g

Sodium: 800 mg
Potassium: 600 mg
Phosphorus: 300 mg

66. Basil Zucchini Spaghetti

Preparation time: 1 hour and 10 minutes

Cooking time: 10 minutes

Servings: 4

Ingredients:

- 1/3 cup coconut oil, melted
- 4 zucchinis, cut with a spiralizer
- 1/4 cup basil, chopped
- A pinch of sea salt
- Black pepper to taste
- 0.25 cup walnuts, chopped
- 2 garlic cloves, minced

Directions:

1. In a bowl, mix zucchini spaghetti with salt and pepper, toss to coat, leave aside for 1 hour, drain well and put in a bowl.

100

2. Warmth up a pan with the oil over medium-high heat, add zucchini spaghetti and garlic, stir and cook for 5 minutes.
3. Add basil and walnuts and black pepper, stir and cook for 3 minutes more.
4. Divide between plates and serve as a side dish
5. Enjoy!

Nutrition Facts Per Serving:

Calories: 287 kcal
Fat: 27 g
Fiber: 3 g
Carbs: 8 g
Protein: 4 g
Sodium: 75 mg
Phosphorus: 110 mg
Potassium: 117 mg

67. Cauliflower Rice and Coconut

Preparation Time: 20 minutes

Cooking Time: 15 minutes

Serving: 4

Ingredients:

- 3 cups cauliflower, riced
- 2/3 cups full-fat coconut milk
- 1-2 teaspoons sriracha paste
- 1/4- 1/2 teaspoon onion powder
- Salt as needed
- Fresh basil for garnish

Directions:

1. Take a pan and place it over medium-low heat.
2. Combine all of the ingredients and stir to mix well.
3. Let cook for about 5-10 minutes, making sure that the lid is on.
4. Then, remove the lid and keep cooking until there's no excess liquid.

5. When the rice becomes creamy, serve it.

Calories: 225
Fat: 19 g
Carbohydrates: 4 g
Protein: 5 g
Sodium: 60 mg
Phosphorus: 150 mg
Potassium: 600 mg

68. Kale and Garlic Platter

Preparation Time: 5 minutes

Cooking Time: 12 minutes

Serving: 2

Ingredients:

- 1/2 bunch kale
- 1 tablespoon olive oil
- 2 garlic cloves, minced

Directions:

1. Remove kale stem and cut into bite-sized pieces.

2. Then, set a large-sized pot and let heat olive oil over medium heat.
3. Add garlic and stir for 2 minutes.
4. Add kale and cook for 5-10 minutes.
5. Serve!

Nutrition Facts Per Serving:

Calories: 121 kcal
Fat: 8 g
Carbohydrates: 5 g
Protein: 4 g
Sodium: 81 mg
Potassium: 900 mg
Phosphorus: 220 mg

69. Healthy, Blistered Beans and Almond

Preparation Time: 10 minutes

Cooking Time: 20 minutes

Serving: 2

Ingredients:

- 1/2 pound fresh green beans, ends trimmed

- 1 tablespoon olive oil
- 1/8 teaspoon salt
- 1 tablespoon fresh dill, minced
- Juice of 1/2 lemon
- 1/8 cup crushed almonds
- Salt as needed

Directions:

1. First, preheat your oven to 400 F.
2. Take a bowl and add in the green beans with olive oil and salt.
3. Then, take a large-sized sheet pan and spread them on it.
4. Roast for 10 minutes and stir nicely, then roast for 8-10 minutes more.
5. Remove it from the oven and keep stirring in the lemon juice alongside the dill.
6. Top it with crushed almonds, some sea salt, and serve.

Nutrition Facts Per Serving:

Calories: 98 kcal

Fat: 7.83 g

Carbohydrates: 7.57 g

Protein: 1.86 g

Sodium: 236 mg

Potassium: 161 mg

Phosphorus: 33 mg

70. Cucumber Soup (Low Caloric)

Preparation Time: 10 minutes

Cooking Time: 0 minutes

Serving: 2

Ingredients:

- 1 tablespoon garlic, minced
- 2 cups English cucumbers, peeled and diced
- 1/4 cup onions, diced
- 1/2 tablespoon lemon juice
- 1 cup vegetable broth
- 1/4 teaspoon salt
- 1/8 teaspoon red pepper flakes
- 1/8 cup parsley, diced
- 1/4 cup Greek yogurt, plain

Directions:

1. Take a blender and attach the listed ingredients (except 1/4 cup of chopped cucumbers).
2. Blend until smooth.
3. Divide the soup amongst four servings and top with extra cucumbers.
4. Serve.

Nutrition Facts Per Serving:

Calories: 53 kcal
Fat: 1.26 g
Carbohydrates: 8.77 g
Protein: 2.33 g
Sodium: 238.19 mg
Potassium: 273 mg
Phosphorus: 67 mg

71. Eggplant Salad

Preparation Time: 10 minutes
Cooking Time: 50 minutes
Serving: 3

Ingredients:

- 2 eggplants, peeled and sliced
- 2 garlic cloves
- 2 green bell pepper, sliced, seeds removed
- 1/2 cup fresh parsley
- 1/2 cup egg-free mayonnaise
- Salt and black pepper

Directions:

1. First, preheat your oven to 480 F.
2. Then, take a baking pan and add the eggplants and bell pepper
3. Bake the vegetables for about 30 minutes and flip them after 20 minutes.
4. Then, take a bowl and add baked vegetables and all the remaining ingredients.
5. Mix well.
6. Serve.

Nutrition Facts Per Serving:

Calories: 196 kcal
Fat: 10.8 g
Carbohydrates: 13.4 g
Protein: 14.6 g
Sodium: 310 mg
Potassium: 1100 mg

Phosphorus: 121 mg

72. Cajun Crab (Low Caloric)

Preparation Time: 10 minutes

Cooking Time: 10 minutes

Serving: 2

Ingredients:

- 1 lemon, fresh and quartered
- 3 tablespoons Cajun seasoning
- 2 bay leaves
- 4 snow crab legs, precooked and defrosted
- 1 tsp. golden ghee

Directions:

1. Set a large pot and fill it about halfway with water and salt.
2. Then, bring the water to a boil.
3. When water is boiling, squeeze the lemon juice into the pot and toss in the remaining lemon quarters.
4. Add bay leaves and Cajun seasoning.
5. Then, season for 1 minute.
6. Add crab legs and boil for about 8 minutes (make sure to keep them submerged the whole time).
7. Melt ghee in the microwave and use it as a dipping sauce.
8. Serve.

Nutrition Facts Per Serving:

Calories: 49.71 kcal
Total Fat: 0.39 g
Carbohydrates: 0.65 g
Protein: 10.39 g
Sodium: 771.66 mg
Potassium: 125.93 mg
Phosphorus: 123 mg

73. Mushroom Pork Chops

Preparation Time: 10 minutes

Cooking Time: 40 minutes

Serving: 3

Ingredients:

- 8 ounces mushrooms, sliced
- 1 teaspoon garlic
- 1 onion, peeled and chopped
- 1 cup egg-free mayonnaise
- 3 pork loins
- 1 teaspoon ground nutmeg
- 1 tablespoon balsamic vinegar
- 1/2 cup of coconut oil

Directions:

1. Take a pan, add the coconut oil and let heat it up over medium heat.
2. Then, add mushrooms, onions, and stir well.
3. Cook for 4 minutes.
4. Add pork loins and season with nutmeg, garlic powder, and let brown both sides.
5. Bring the pan to the oven and bake for 30 minutes at 350 F.
6. Transfer pork loins to plates and place aluminum foil on top to keep them warm.
7. Take the same pan and place it over medium heat.
8. Add vinegar, mayonnaise over the mushroom mixture and stir for a few minutes.
9. Drizzle sauce over pork loins.
10. Serve.

Nutrition Facts Per Serving:

Calories: 400 kcal
Total Fat: 18.39 g
Carbohydrates: 1.4 g
Protein: 30g
Sodium: 91.71 mg
Potassium: 158.89 mg
Phosphorus: 73.72 mg

74. Caramelized Pork Chops

Preparation Time: 5 minutes

Cooking Time: 30 minutes

Serving: 2

Ingredients:

- 2 pounds pork chops
- 1 tsp. salt
- 1 tsp. pepper
- ½ tsp. olive oil
- 2 ounces green chili, chopped
- 2 tablespoons chili powder
- 1/4 teaspoon dried oregano
- 1/4 teaspoon ground cumin
- 1 garlic clove, minced
- 1 onion, sliced
- ½ glass of water

Directions:

1. Coat your pork chops with 1/2 teaspoon of pepper and 1/2 teaspoon of seasoning salt, chili powder, oregano and cumin.
2. Then, take a skillet and heat 1/2 tsp. oil over medium heat with the garlic.
3. Brown your pork chops on each side.
4. Add water and onion to the skillet.
5. Cover and lower the heat, simmer it for about 20 minutes.
6. Turn your loins over and add the rest of the pepper and salt.
7. Cover until the water evaporates and the onions turn a medium brown texture.
8. Remove the chops from your skillet.
9. Serve with some onions on top!

Nutrition Facts Per Serving:

Calories: 500 kcal

Fat: 19 g

Carbohydrates: 4 g

Protein: 27 g

Sodium: 91.71 mg

Potassium: 153.89 mg

Phosphorus: 73.72 mg

75. Mediterranean Pork

Preparation Time: 10 minutes

Cooking Time: 35 minutes

Serving: 2

Ingredients:

- 2 pork chops, bone-in
- ½ tsp. salt
- pepper to taste
- 1/2 teaspoon dried rosemary
- 1 1/2 garlic cloves, peeled and minced

Directions:

1. First, preheat your oven to 425 F.
2. Season pork chops with salt and pepper.
3. Place them in a roasting pan and add rosemary and garlic.
4. Bake for 10 minutes.

5. Lower heat to 350 ° F and roast for 25 minutes more.
6. Slice pork chops and divide on plates.
7. Drizzle pan juice all over
8. Serve.

Nutrition Facts Per Serving:

Calories: 335 kcal

Fat: 17.42 g

Carbohydrates: 1.52 g

Protein: 40.48 g

Sodium: 668 mg

Potassium: 566 mg

Phosphorus: 351 mg

76. Ground Beef and Bell Peppers

Preparation Time: 10 minutes

Cooking Time: 10 minutes

Serving: 2

Ingredients:

- 1 onion, chopped
- 1 tablespoon coconut oil
- 0.5 pound ground beef
- 1 red bell pepper, diced

- 1 cup spinach, chopped
- ¼ tsp. salt
- ¼ tsp. black pepper

Directions:

1. Take a skillet, add coconut oil and onion and let them cook over medium-high heat until the onion is lightly browned.
2. Then, add spinach, salt, and ground beef.
3. Stir fry until done.
4. Meanwhile, clean the inside of the red bell pepper by eliminating all the seeds.
5. Then, take the mixture from the skillet and fill up the bell pepper.
6. Serve.

Nutrition Facts Per Serving:

Calories: 337 kcal
Fat: 19.61 g
Carbohydrates: 7.89 g
Protein: 31.68 g
Potassium: 581 mg
Sodium: 376 mg

Phosphorus: 252 mg

77. Spiced Up Pork Chops

Preparation Time: 4 hours
Cooking Time: 14 minutes
Serving: 4

Ingredients:

- 1/4 cup lime juice
- 4 pork rib chops
- 1 tablespoon coconut oil, melted
- 2 garlic cloves, peeled and minced
- 1 tablespoon chili powder
- 1 teaspoon ground cinnamon
- 2 teaspoons cumin
- Salt and pepper to taste
- 1/2 teaspoon hot pepper sauce
- 1 Mango, sliced

Directions:

1. Combine lime juice, oil, garlic, cumin, cinnamon, chili powder, salt, pepper,

hot pepper sauce in a bowl and whisk well.

2. Then, add pork chops and toss.

3. Keep it on the side and refrigerate for 4 hours.

4. Preheat your grill to medium heat and transfer pork chops to it.

5. Grill for 7 minutes per side.

6. Divide between serving platters and serve with mango slices.

Nutrition Facts Per Serving:

Calories: 400 kcal

Fat: 8 g

Carbohydrates: 3 g

Protein: 35 g

Sodium: 91.71 mg

Potassium: 153.89 mg

Phosphorus: 73.72 mg

78. Healthy, Juicy Salmon Dish

Note: To make this recipe, you need a pot with "Sauté Mode", like an Instant Pot or others, if you prefer.

| Preparation Time: 5 minutes |
| Cooking Time: 13 minutes |
| Serving: 1 |

Ingredients:

- 1/4 cup of water
- Few sprigs of parsley, basil, tarragon
- 0.5 pound of salmon, skin on
- 1 teaspoon of ghee
- 1 tbsp. + 1 tsp. teaspoon of salt
- 2 tbsp. + 2 tsp. of pepper
- 1/4 of lemon, thinly sliced
- 0.5 whole carrot, julienned

Directions:

1. Set your pot to Sauté mode and add water and herbs.

2. Place a steamer rack inside your pot and place salmon.

3. Drizzle ghee on top of the salmon and season with salt and pepper.

110

4. Cover with lemon slices.
5. Lock the lid of the pot and cook on HIGH pressure for 3 minutes.
6. Release the pressure naturally over 10 minutes.
7. Transfer the salmon to a serving platter.
8. Set your pot to Sauté mode and add carrots with parsley, basil and tarragon.
9. Cook for 1-2 minutes and transfer to the platter with salmon.
10. Serve.

Nutrition Facts Per Serving:

Calories: 464 kcal
Fat: 34 g
Carbohydrates: 3 g
Protein: 34 g
Sodium: 424 mg
Potassium: 984.18 mg
Phosphorus: 488.19 mg

79. Platter-o-Brussels

Preparation Time: 10 minutes
Cooking Time: 25 minutes
Serving: 2

Ingredients:

- 1 tablespoon olive oil
- 1/2 yellow onion, chopped
- 1 pound Brussels sprouts, trimmed and halved
- 2 cups chicken stock
- 1/2 tsp. black pepper
- 1/8 cup coconut cream

Directions:

1. Take a pot and let the oil heat up over medium heat.
2. Add onion and stir to cook for 3 minutes.
3. Add Brussels sprouts and stir, cook for 2 minutes.
4. Then, add stock and black pepper, stir and bring to a simmer.
5. Cook for 20 minutes more.

6. Now, with an immersion blender, make the soup creamy.
7. Add coconut cream and stir well.
8. Ladle into soup bowls and serve.

Nutrition Facts Per Serving:

Calories 621.97kcal
Total Fat 26.29g
Carbs 78.24g
Sugars 33.01g
Protein 28.23g
Sodium 811.43mg
Potassium 2000mg
Phosphorus 400mg

80. Almond Chicken

Preparation Time: 15 minutes
Cooking Time: 15 minutes
Serving: 3

Ingredients:

- 2 large chicken breasts, boneless and skinless
- 1/3 cup lemon juice
- 1 1/2 cups seasoned almond meal
- 2 tablespoons coconut oil
- Lemon pepper, to taste
- Parsley for decoration

Directions:

1. Cut chicken breasts in half and slice each half until 1/4 inch thick.
2. Take a pan and let heat up the oil over medium heat.
3. Dip each chicken breast slice into lemon juice and let it sit for 2 minutes.
4. Turnover and let the other side sit for 2 minutes as well.
5. Then, transfer to almond meal and coat both sides.
6. Attach coated chicken to the oil and fry for 4 minutes per side, making sure to sprinkle lemon pepper liberally.
7. Transfer to a paper-lined sheet and repeat until all chicken is fried.
8. Garnish with parsley and serve.

Nutrition Facts Per Serving:

Calories: 360kcal

Fat: 24g

Carbohydrates: 3g

Protein: 44g

Sodium 84mg

Potassium 707mg

Phosphorus 400mg

81. Blackberry Chicken Wings

Prep Time: 35 minutes

Cook Time: 45 minutes

Serving: 2

Ingredients:

- 0.75 pounds chicken wings, about 20 pieces
- 1/4 cup blackberry chipotle jam
- Salt and pepper to taste
- 1/4 cup of water

Directions:

1. Take a bowl, add water and jam and mix well to make the marinade.

2. Now, place chicken wings in a zip bag and add two-thirds of the marinade.

3. Then, season with salt and pepper.

4. Let it marinate for 30 minutes.

5. Meanwhile, preheat your oven to 400°F.

6. Prepare a baking sheet, place chicken wings on it, and bake for 15 minutes.

7. After this time, brush the remaining marinade and bake for 30 minutes more.

8. Serve.

Nutrition Facts Per Serving:

Calories: 702kcal

Fat: 29g

Carbohydrates: 01.8g

Protein: 45g

Sodium 600mg

Potassium 400mg

Phosphorus 200mg

82. Fennel and Figs Lamb

Prep Time: 10 minutes
Cook Time: 40 minutes
Serving: 2

Ingredients:

- 6 ounces lamb racks
- 1 fennel bulb, sliced
- Salt and pepper to taste
- 1 tablespoon olive oil
- 2 figs, cut in half
- 1/8 cup apple cider vinegar
- 1/2 tablespoon swerve

Directions:

1. Mix the fennel, figs, vinegar, swerve, and oil in a bowl and toss.
2. Then, transfer to a baking dish and season with salt and pepper.
3. Bake for 15 minutes at 400 F.
4. Meanwhile, spread salt and pepper over the lamb and transfer to a heated pan over medium-high heat.
5. Cook for about 5 minutes.
6. Add lamb to the baking dish with fennel and bake for 20 minutes.
7. Divide between plates and serve.

Nutrition Facts Per Serving:

Calories: 456.76 kcal
Total Fat: 31.02 g
Carbohydrates: 28.63 g
Protein: 23.02 g
Sodium: 410.1 mg
Potassium: 1126.45
Phosphorus: 257.76 mg

83. Herbed Butter Pork Chops

Preparation Time: 5 minutes
Cooking Time: 25 minutes
Serving: 2

Ingredients:

- 1 tablespoon almond butter, divided
- 2 boneless pork chops

- Salt and pepper to taste
- 1 tablespoon dried Italian seasoning
- 1 tablespoon olive oil

Directions:

1. First, preheat your oven to 350 F.
2. Take pork chops and dry them with a paper towel. Then, place them in a baking dish.
3. Season with salt, pepper, and Italian seasoning.
4. Drizzle olive oil over pork chops and top each chop with 1/2 tablespoon butter.
5. Bake for 25 minutes.
6. Transfer pork chops onto two plates and top with butter juice.
7. Serve.

Nutrition Facts Per Serving:

Calories: 333 kcal
Fat: 23 g
Carbohydrates: 1 g
Protein: 31g
Sodium: 91.71 mg

Potassium: 153.89 mg
Phosphorus: 73.72 mg

84. Simple Rice Mushroom Risotto

Prep Time: 5 minutes
Cook Time: 15 minutes
Serving: 2

Ingredients:

- 2 1/2 cups cauliflower, riced
- 1 1/2 tablespoon coconut oil
- 1/2 pound Portobello mushrooms, thinly sliced
- 1/2 pound white mushrooms, thinly sliced
- 1 shallot, diced
- 1/8 cup organic vegetable broth
- Salt and pepper to taste
- 1 1/2 tablespoons chives, chopped
- 2 tablespoons almond butter

Directions:

1. Using a food processor, blend cauliflower florets until riced.
2. Then, take a large saucepan and heat 1/2 tablespoons coconut oil over medium-high flame.
3. Add mushrooms and sauté for 3 minutes; mushrooms must be tender.
4. Remove the mushrooms from the saucepan, along with the liquid, and keep them on the side.
5. Add the rest of the 1 tablespoon coconut oil to the skillet and let heat it.
6. Toss shallot and cook for 60 seconds.
7. Add cauliflower rice, stir for 2 minutes until coated with oil.
8. Add broth to riced cauliflower and stir for 5 minutes.
9. Remove skillet from heat and mix in mushrooms and liquid.
10. Add chives, butter and season with salt and pepper
11. Serve.

Nutrition Facts Per Serving:

Calories: 555.21kcal
Total Fat 39.91g
Carbs: 38.14g
Sugars: 18g
Protein: 26.16g
Sodium: 640mg
Potassium: 2500mg
Phosphorus: 640mg

85. Zucchini Bowl

Preparation Time: 10 minutes

Cooking Time: 25 minutes

Serving: 2

Ingredients:

- 1/2 onion, chopped
- 2 zucchini, cut into medium chunks
- 1 tablespoon coconut milk
- 1 garlic clove, minced

116

- 2 cups chicken stock
- 1 tablespoon coconut oil
- Pinch of salt
- Black pepper to taste

Directions:

1. Take a pot and let heat the oil over medium heat.
2. Add zucchini, garlic, onion, and stir—Cook for 5 minutes.
3. Add stock, salt, pepper, and stir.
4. Set to a boil, and then lower down the heat.
5. Simmer for 20 minutes.
6. Turn off the heat and add coconut milk.
7. Use an immersion blender until smooth.
8. Pour into soup bowls and serve.

Nutrition Facts Per Serving:

Calories: 404.35 kcal
Total Fat: 23.86 g
Carbohydrates: 33.37 g
Protein: 16.84 g
Sodium: 787.77 mg
Potassium: 1409.78 mg

Phosphorus: 277.65 mg

86. Nice Coconut Haddock (Healthy, Low Caloric)

Preparation Time: 10 minutes

Cooking Time: 12 minutes

Serving: 3

Ingredients:

- 4 haddock fillets, 5 ounces each, boneless
- 2 tablespoons coconut oil, melted
- 1 cup coconut, shredded and unsweetened
- 1/4 cup hazelnuts, ground
- Salt to taste

Directions:

1. First, preheat your oven to 400 F.
2. Then, line a baking sheet with parchment paper and keep it on the side.

3. Take a bowl and stir in hazelnuts and shredded coconut.
4. Then, pat fish fillets with a paper towel, season with salt and drag them through the coconut mix until both sides are coated well.
5. Transfer the fish fillets to the baking sheet and brush them with coconut oil.
6. Bake for about 12 minutes until flaky.
7. Serve.

Nutrition Facts Per Serving:

Calories: 192 kcal
Total Fat: 16.24 g
Carbohydrates: 4.85 g
Protein: 8.43 g
Sodium: 165 mg
Potassium: 385 mg
Phosphorus: 134 mg

Dinner

87. Healthy Steamed Fish

Preparation time: 10 minutes

Cooking time: 25 minutes

Servings: 2

Ingredients:

- 1/4 cup olive oil
- 2 fillets of tilapia
- 1/4 cup onion, sliced
- 6 tbsp. red and green peppers, sliced
- 1/2 tsp. hot pepper sauce
- 1/8 tsp. black pepper
- 1/2 tbsp Ketchup
- 1/2 large sprig thyme
- 1/2 cup hot water
- 1/2 tbsp lime juice

Directions:

1. Take a frying pan and warm the oil on medium.
2. Sauté bell peppers and onion.
3. Add 1/4 cup of hot water along with lime juice, ketchup, thyme, hot pepper sauce, and black pepper. Stir.
4. Now, put fish in the pan.
5. Add 1/4 cup of hot water. Spoon veggies and sauce over fish.
6. Cook for 5 minutes with the lid on.
7. Then, turn fish and keep cooking covered until done.

Nutrition Facts Per Serving:

Calories: 764.13 kcal

Total Fat: 61.11 g

Protein: 47.64 g

Carbohydrates: 9.27 g

Sodium: 267.81 mg

Potassium: 835 mg

Phosphorus: 430 mg

88. Broiled Salmon in Maple

Preparation time: 2 hours

Cooking time: 30 minutes

Servings: 4

Ingredients:

- 3 tbsp. maple syrup
- 1 lb. salmon fillets

- 1 tbsp. low sodium soy sauce
- 3 tbsp. lemon juice
- 2 tbsp. fresh cilantro
- 2 garlic cloves, pressed
- 1 tbsp. green onion, chopped

Directions:

1. To form a marinade, take a bowl and add all the ingredients, except salmon.
2. Then, put salmon fillets on a platter and pour marinade over them. Leave the salmon marinating for 2 hours, covered in the fridge.
3. Preheat a grill pan over medium-high for about 2 minutes and cook the salmon on each side for 4-5 minutes, after removing it from the marinade.
4. Serve the salmon hot or cold, as you prefer, with a wedge of salmon.

Nutrition Facts Per Serving:

Protein: 23 g
Carbohydrates: 12 g
Fat: 7 g
Calories: 340 kcal
Sodium: 75 mg
Potassium: 600 mg
Phosphorus: 350 mg

89. Chickpea Curry and Eggplant (Vegetarian)

Preparation time: 15 minutes

Cooking time: 40 minutes

Servings: 3

Ingredients:

- 1 tbsp. sunflower oil
- 1 small eggplant
- 5-6 curry leaves
- 1/2 tbsp. brown or black mustard seeds
- 1 dried chili, chopped
- 1 onion, finely chopped
- 1 tsp. ground coriander
- 2 tsp. garam masala
- 1 tsp. turmeric

- 1/2 cup reduced-sodium vegetable broth
- 1/2 cup of water
- 1 1/2 tomatoes, quartered
- 1/2 cup yogurt, plain, low fat
- 1 cup of canned chickpeas

Directions:

1. Cut the eggplant in half and reduce it into medium-sized wedges.
2. Take a large pan, warm up 1/4 tbsp oil and cook the eggplant wedges for 3 minutes until crispy and brown. Put them aside on a plate.
3. Then, in the same pan, add curry leaves, mustard seeds, and remaining oil to the pan. Keep cooking for 30 seconds.
4. Now, stir in the onion, cooking until it begins to brown and soften.
5. Add spices and the dried chili, cook for 1 minute.
6. Add 1/2 cup vegetable broth, 1/2 cup of water, 1/2 cup of yogurt, and tomatoes. Simmer for 30 minutes until saucy and thick.
7. Stir in eggplant and chickpeas. Simmer for 5 minutes until eggplants are tender and everything is hot.
8. Serve with warm naan bread or rice with curry leaves, if you like.

Nutrition Facts Per Serving:

Calories: 335.64 kcal
Protein 12.59 g
Carbohydrates: 47.09 g
Total Fat: 13.25 gg
Sodium: 486.31
Potassium: 1136.14 mg
Phosphorus: 260 mg

90. Curried Veggies and Rice

Preparation Time: 12 minutes

Cooking Time: 25 minutes

Servings: 4

Ingredients:

- 1/4 cup olive oil
- 0.5 cup long-grain white basmati rice
- 4 garlic cloves, minced
- 2 1/2 tsp. curry powder
- 1 cup sliced shiitake mushrooms
- 1 red bell pepper, chopped
- 1 cup frozen, shelled edamame
- 2 cups low-sodium vegetable broth
- 1/8 tsp. freshly ground black pepper

Directions:

1. Take a large pot, and heat the olive oil on medium heat.
2. Then, add the rice, garlic, curry powder, mushrooms, bell pepper, and edamame.
3. Cook, stirring for 3 minutes.
4. Add the broth and black pepper and bring to a boil.
5. Reduce the heat to low, partially cover the pot, and simmer for 15–18 minutes or until the rice is tender. Stir and serve.

Nutrition Facts Per Serving:

Calories: 347kcal

Fats: 16 g

Carbs: 44 g

Protein: 8 g

Sodium: 114 mg

Phosphorus: 131 mg

Potassium: 334 mg

91. Chickpea Bites and Eggplant (Low Caloric, Vegetarian)

Preparation time: 10 minutes

Cooking time: 60 minutes

Servings: 20

Ingredients:

- 3 large eggplants, halved
- 2 tsp. cumin seeds
- 2 tsp. coriander
- 2 large garlic cloves, peeled
- 2 cups canned chickpeas, drained and rinsed
- 1/2 lemon zested and juice
- 2 tbsp. chickpea flour
- 3 tbsp polenta
- 1/2 lemon

Directions:

1. First, preheat the oven to 356 F.
2. Spray the eggplant halves with cooking spray. Put them cut side up in a large roasting pan and season with the cumin seeds, coriander, and garlic.
3. Roast for 40 minutes until the eggplant will be completely tender.
4. Scoop the eggplant flesh into a bowl. Discard the skins.
5. With a spatula, mix in the garlic and spices. Add lemon juice and zest, chickpea flour, and chickpeas. Mash together.
6. Shape the mixture into 20 balls. Set the balls on a baking tray that is lined with baking parchment. Chill for 30 minutes in the fridge.
7. Sprinkle polenta on a plate. Roll the balls in it to coat. Return them to the tray. Spray each one with a little oil. Roast for 20 minutes until golden, hot, and crispy. Serve with lemon wedges.

Calories: 89.47 kcal
Total Fat: 1.38 g
Protein: 4.09 g
Carbohydrates: 16.84 g
Sodium: 138.82 mg
Potassium: 343.15 mg
Phosphorus: 71 mg

92. Sesame Asparagus (Healthy, Low Caloric)

Preparation time: 5 minutes

Cooking time: 15 minutes

Servings: 2

Ingredients:

- 1/2 tbsp. lemon juice
- 8 asparagus spears
- 1/2 tsp. sesame seeds
- 1 tbsp. sesame oil

Directions:

1. First, preheat the oven at 375 F.

2. Take a bowl and mix asparagus with sesame seeds, lemon juice, and sesame oil.

3. Wrap the asparagus in tinfoil, and bake them in the preheated oven for about 15 minutes or until tender.

Nutrition Facts Per Serving:

Calories: 68 kcal
Protein: 2 g
Carbohydrates: 4 g
Fat: 0.4 g
Sodium: 1 mg
Potassium: 35 mg
Phosphorus: 12 mg

93. Chicken Bacon Wraps

Preparation Time: 10 minutes

Cooking time: 20 minutes

Servings: 4

Ingredients:

- 2 chicken breasts, boneless, skinless

- 4 slices bacon, hick-cut
- 1/4 cup brown Swerve
- 2 teaspoons smoked paprika
- 1/2 teaspoon garlic powder
- 1/4 teaspoon onion powder
- 1/2 teaspoon black pepper

Directions:

1. Cover each chicken breast with 2 bacon slices and place them in a baking pan.
2. Whisk the Swerve with all the spices and drizzle over the wrapped chicken.
3. Spray the chicken with cooking oil.
4. Bake at 350 degrees F.
5. Slice and serve.

Nutrition Facts Per Serving:

Calories: 611.54 kcal
Total Fat: 41.17 g
Cholesterol: 92 mg
Sodium: 475.59 mg
Carbohydrate: 1.7 g

Sugars: 0.3 g
Protein: 54.2 g
Phosphorous: 2440 mg
Potassium: 600 mg

94. Rosemary and Roasted Cauliflower (Healthy, Low Caloric)

Preparation time: 10 minutes

Cooking time: 30 minutes

Servings: 9

Ingredients:

- 1 1/2 tablespoons olive oil
- 1 medium head cauliflower
- 1/4 teaspoon salt
- 1 tbsp. fresh rosemary, finely chopped
- Fresh ground black pepper

Directions:

1. First, preheat the oven to 450F.
2. Then, remove florets from the cauliflower head and cut it into bite-size pieces.
3. Take a large bowl, and pitch the cauliflower with the rest of the ingredients.
4. Spread the seasoned cauliflower on an ungreased baking sheet.
5. Roast for 15 minutes. Remove from the oven and stir.
6. Cook until the cauliflower is tender.

Nutrition Facts Per Serving:

Calories: 30 kcal
Protein: 1 g
Carbohydrates: 2 g
Fat: 2.36 g
Sodium: 74 mg
Phosphorus: 13 mg
Potassium: 93 mg

95. Shrimp with Salsa

Preparation Time: 15 minutes

Cooking Time: 10 minutes

Servings: 4

Ingredients:

- Olive oil 2 Tbsp.
- Large shrimp 6 ounces, peeled and deveined, tails left on
- Minced garlic 1 tsp.
- Chopped English cucumber 1/2 cup
- Chopped mango 1/2 cup
- Zest of 1 lime
- Juice of 1 lime
- Ground black pepper
- Lime wedges for garnish

Directions:

1. Take four wooden skewers and rinse them in water for 30 minutes.
2. After that, preheat the barbecue over medium heat.

3. Take a bowl and combine the olive oil, shrimp, and garlic and mix well.
4. Insert the shrimp into the skewers, about four shrimp per skewer.
5. Next, take a bowl and mix the mango, cucumber, lime zest, lime juice, and pepper. Set aside.
6. At this point, grill the shrimp for 10 minutes, turning once or until the shrimp are cooked through.
7. Season shrimp lightly with pepper.
8. Arrange cucumber sauce on plates and place shrimp on top with lime wedges on the sides. Serve.

Nutrition Facts Per Serving:

Calories: 220 kcal
Fat: 15.08 g
Carbs: 5.91 g
Sugars: 4.07 g
Phosphorus: 196 mg
Potassium: 316 mg

Sodium: 480.36 mg
Protein: 12.5 g

96. Green Bean Garlic Salad (Healthy, Low Caloric)

Preparation time: 5 minutes

Cooking time: 20 minutes

Servings: 2

Ingredients:

- 1 clove garlic, chopped
- 1 cup green beans
- 1/2 tbsp. sesame oil
- 1/2 tbsp. balsamic or red wine vinegar

Directions:

1. First, clean the beans. Then, take a medium pot and set some water to boil.
2. Cook them in boiling water until tender.
3. Drain and cool them under cold water.

4. Pitch the beans with oil, vinegar, and garlic.

Calories: 50 kcal
Protein: 1 g
Carbohydrates: 6 g
Fat: 4 g
Sodium: 2 mg
Phosphorus: 18 mg
Potassium: 81 mg

97. Ginger Cauliflower Rice

Preparation time: 10 minutes
Cooking time: 10 minutes
Servings: 4

Ingredients:

- 5 cups cauliflower florets
- 3 tablespoons coconut oil
- 4 ginger slices, grated
- 1 tablespoon coconut vinegar
- 3 garlic cloves, minced
- 1 tablespoon chives, minced
- 0.5-1 tsp of sea salt
- Black pepper to taste

Directions:

1. Set cauliflower florets in a food processor and pulse well.
2. Warmth up a pan with the oil over medium-high heat, add ginger, stir and cook for 3 minutes.
3. Add cauliflower rice and garlic, stir and cook for 7 minutes.
4. Add salt, black pepper, vinegar, and chives, stir, cook for a few seconds more, divide between plates and serve.
5. Enjoy!

Nutrition Facts Per Serving:

Calories: 125 kcal
Fat: 10.4 g
Fiber: 12 g
Carbs: 7 g
Protein: 2 g
Phosphorus: 110 mg
Potassium: 117 mg
Sodium: 75 mg

98. Asparagus Fried Rice

Preparation Time: 10 minutes

Cooking Time: 15 minutes

Servings: 1

Ingredients:

- 2 medium eggs, beaten
- 1/2 tsp. ground ginger
- 2 tsps. low-sodium soy sauce
- 2 tbsps. olive oil
- 1 onion, chopped
- 4 garlic cloves, minced
- 1 cup sliced cremini mushrooms
- 5 oz. white rice, thawed
- 8 oz. fresh asparagus, about 15 spears, cut into 1-inch pieces

Directions:

1. Take a small bowl and whisk the eggs, along with the ginger, and soy sauce and set aside.
2. Heat the olive oil in a medium skillet or wok over medium heat.
3. Add the onion and garlic and sauté for 2 minutes until tender-crisp.
4. Add the mushrooms and rice, and stir-fry for 3 minutes longer.
5. Put asparagus and cook for 2–3 minutes.
6. Pour in the egg mixture. Stir the eggs until cooked through, about 2–3 minutes, and stir into the rice mixture.
7. Serve.

Nutrition Facts Per Serving:

Calories: 490 kcal

Fats: 13 g

Carbs: 25 g

Protein: 9 g

Sodium: 600 mg

Potassium: 530 mg

Phosphorus: 211 mg

99. Shrimp Spaghetti

Preparation time: 10 minutes

Cooking time: 30 minutes

Servings: 4

Ingredients:

- 1/3 cup extra virgin olive oil
- 1/2 lb. spaghetti or spaghettini
- 1/4 tsp. crushed red chilies
- 2 cloves garlic, crushed
- 1 red pepper, diced
- 1 lb. raw shrimp
- 1/3 cup dry white wine
- 1/3 cup toasted fresh breadcrumbs
- Chopped fresh parsley (optional)
- Freshly ground pepper, to taste

Direction:

1. First, take a medium-size pot and put some water to boil to cook pasta.
2. Meanwhile, take a large skillet, and warm up the oil over medium-low.
3. Add crushed red chilies and garlic - Cook, stirring, for 1 minute.
4. Add pepper, cooking for 5 minutes.
5. Add the shrimp. Cook for 1 minute.
6. Add the wine.
7. Turn the heat up to medium. Simmer until the shrimp start to curl and turn opaque.
8. Drain pasta. Put it in a large serving dish.
9. Pour sauce over pasta. Toss together with breadcrumbs.
10. Serve with parsley and freshly ground pepper.

Nutrition Facts Per Serving:

Calories: 299 kcal
Protein: 29.24 g
Carbohydrates 19.17 g
Total Fat: 11.75 g
Sodium: 1315 mg
Potassium: 263 mg

Phosphorus: 332 mg

100. Pork Pineapple Roast

Note: this recipe is prepared by using a Crock-Pot. In alternatives, you can use other types of slow cooker or any heavy-duty pot with a decent cover in a low temp oven (after boiling first) or even a Dutch oven. Choose what you prefer.

Preparation time: 7 minutes

Cooking time: 6 hours

Servings: 3

Ingredients:

- 1/2 tbsp. black pepper
- 1/2 (1 lb.) pork roast
- 1/2 (4 oz.) can crushed pineapple
- 1 tbsp. sugar or Splenda
- 1/4 tsp. crushed red chilies
- 1/2 clove garlic, minced
- 1/4 tbsp. low-sodium soy sauce
- 1 tbsp. cornstarch
- 1/8 tsp. dried basil
- 1/2 green or red pepper, chopped
- 1/8 cup cold water

Directions:

1. Cut roast in half. Put it in the Crock-Pot.
2. Combine all ingredients except green pepper, water, and cornstarch. Pour over roast. Cover it and cook for 4-6 hours on high.
3. Remove roast. Ensure the internal temperature is 170 F.
4. Drain pineapple, reserving liquid. Return pineapple and meat to the cooker.
5. Add water to pineapple liquid to make 1 3/4 cups.
6. Blend cold water and cornstarch to form a smooth paste. Stir into hot reserved liquid.
7. Add chopped red and green pepper.
8. Cook until thickened.

Nutrition Facts Per Serving:

Calories: 958.79 kcal
Protein: 80.25 g
Carbohydrates: 28.99 g
Total Fat: 56.34 g
Sodium: 352.61 mg
Potassium: 1700 mg
Phosphorus: 890 mg

101. Curry Pork Lime Kebabs

Preparation time: 1 hour

Cooking time: 15 minutes

Servings: 2

Ingredients:

- 1 tbsp. chopped fresh parsley or cilantro
- 1 tbsp. lime juice
- 1/2 tbsp. olive oil
- 1/2 tbsp. packed brown sugar
- 1/4 tsp. of grated lime rind
- 1 tsp. curry powder
- Pinch of pepper
- 1/8 teaspoon salt
- 1/2 large green or red pepper
- 1/2 pork tenderloin

Directions:

1. Take 2 wooden skewers and soak them in water for 30 minutes.
2. Cut pork into 1/2 inch cubes.
3. Whip together the first 8 ingredients, adding pork. Toss to coat.
4. Cover and marinate for 30 minutes.
5. Cut pepper into chunks.
6. Thread pepper chunks and pork onto each skewer.
7. Grill at medium heat for 15 minutes.

Nutrition Facts Per Serving:

Calories: 860 kcal
Protein 65 g
Carbohydrates: 7g
Fat: 5g
Sodium: 352.61
Potassium: 1700 mg
Phosphorus: 890 mg

102. Beef Salad (Healthy)

Preparation time: 15 minutes

Cooking time: 35 minutes

Servings: 6

Ingredients:

- 4 cups torn romaine lettuce
- 1/4 cup each julienned cucumber, sweet yellow pepper, and red onion
- 2 tsp. canola oil
- 1/4 cup of halved grape tomatoes
- 1/2 lb. Beef Strip Loin
- 1/2 tbsp. minced ginger root
- 1/2 tbsp. fresh lime juice
- 1/2 tbsp. cornstarch
- 1/2 tsp. sesame oil
- 1/2 tsp. Asian chili sauce
- 1 clove garlic, minced

For Chili-Lime Vinaigrette:

- 1/4 cup fresh lime juice
- 1 tsp. of grated lime rind
- 1 tbsp. sodium-reduced soy sauce
- 1 tbsp. honey
- 1 tbsp. Asian chili sauce
- 2 tbsp. rice vinegar

Directions:

1. Take a medium bowl and combine the chili sauce, sesame oil, garlic, lime juice, ginger root, and cornstarch.
2. Add beef. Toss to coat. Let stand for 10 minutes.
3. Take a large frypan and warmth 1 tsp. canola oil.
4. Then, stir-fry onion, yellow pepper, cucumber, tomatoes until just wilted and hot. Transfer to the clean bowl.
5. Now, heat the remaining canola oil in the same pan. Stir-fry beef until cooked and browned.
6. Add to wilted vegetables, tossing to combine. Whisk all Chili-Lime Vinaigrette ingredients together.
7. Put Chili-Lime Vinaigrette in the pan. Cook until hot and slightly thickened.

8. Put veggies, beef, and vinaigrette over romaine lettuce and serve.

Nutrition Facts Per Serving:

Calories: 346.07 kcal
Total Fat: 19.31 g
Protein: 26.69 g
Carbohydrates: 16.91 g
Sodium: 312.39 mg
Potassium: 912 mg
Phosphorus: 56 mg

103. Chicken Stew with Kale and Mushrooms

Preparation time: 5 minutes
Cooking time: 35 minutes
Servings: 4

Ingredients

- 1 clove garlic, minced
- 1/4 cup onion, diced
- 1/2 cup shiitake mushrooms, washed, stemmed, and sliced
- 1/2 cup red pepper, chopped
- 1 cup kale, washed, stemmed, and chopped
- 1/2 cup button mushrooms, washed, stemmed and sliced
- 2 cups cooked chicken (or turkey), chopped
- 1 tbsp. olive oil
- 1/2 tbsp. poultry seasoning
- 2 cups no salt added or homemade chicken stock
- 1/4 tsp. garlic powder
- 1/2 tsp. paprika
- 1 tsp. cornstarch
- 1/2 tsp. ground black pepper
- 1/2 cup milk

Directions:

1. Take a large skillet and sauté garlic and onion, until the onion becomes soft and translucent.
2. Then, add remaining veggies and cook until they become brown.

3. Add dry spices, chicken stock, and cooked chicken to veggie mixture. Bring to a simmer.
4. Now, combine milk and cornstarch in a separate container. Stir into the stew.
5. As soon as the stew has thickened, it is ready to serve.

Nutrition Facts Per Serving:

Calories: 337 kcal
Protein 13.86 g
Carbohydrates 8.6 g
Fat 27.69 g
Sodium: 54 mg
Phosphorus: 126 mg
Potassium: 270 mg

104. Egg and Veggie Fajitas

Preparation Time: 15 minutes
Cooking Time: 10 minutes
Servings: 4

Ingredients:

- 1 medium egg
- 3 egg whites
- 2 tsps. chili powder
- 1 tbsp. unsalted butter
- 1 onion, chopped
- 2 garlic cloves, minced
- 1 jalapeño pepper, minced
- 1 red bell pepper, chopped
- 1 cup frozen corn, thawed and drained
- 3 (6-inch) corn tortillas

Directions:

1. Take a small bowl and whisk the egg, egg whites, and chili powder, until well-combined. Then, set aside.
2. Now, melt the butter in a large skillet on medium heat.

136

3. Sauté the onion, garlic, jalapeño, bell pepper, and corn until the vegetables are tender, about 3–4 minutes.
4. Add the beaten egg mixture to the skillet. Cook, occasionally stirring, until the eggs form large curds and are set, about 3–5 minutes.
5. Meanwhile, soften the corn tortillas as directed on the package.
6. Divide the egg mixture evenly among the softened corn tortillas. Roll the tortillas up and serve.

Nutrition Facts Per Serving:

Calories: 450 kcal
Fats: 14 g
Carbs: 35 g
Protein: 14 g
Sodium: 167 mg
Potassium: 408 mg
Phosphorus: 287 mg

105. Healthy Rice and Chicken Soup

Preparation time: 7 minutes
Cooking time: 30 minutes
Servings: 4

Ingredients:

- 1/2 cup white onion, finely chopped
- 1/2 cup celery, diced
- 1 tbsp. Extra virgin oil
- 1/2 cup baby carrots, chopped
- 1/4 tsp. fresh ground black pepper
- 6 tbsps. instant white rice
- 1/2 bay leaf
- 2 fresh thyme sprigs
- 1 boneless skinless chicken breast half
- 3 cups unsalted added chicken/vegetable broth
- 1 tbsp. lime juice

Directions:

1. Take a large pot and sauté celery, carrot, and onion

137

in olive oil. Cook until softened.

2. Then, cook rice.
3. Add pepper, fresh thyme, bay leaf, rice, and stock to the pot and bring to a boil.
4. Set heat and let simmer for 15 minutes.
5. Add chicken and cook ten minutes more.
6. Add lime juice.
7. Remove bay leaf before serving.

Nutrition Facts Per Serving:

Calories 224 kcal
Protein 17.67 g
Carbohydrates 25.88 g
Fat 5.9 g
Sodium: 88 mg
Potassium: 500 mg
Phosphorus: 208 mg

106. Healthy Panini

Preparation time: 15 minutes

Cooking time: 10 minutes

Servings: 2

Ingredients:

- 1 1/2 tbsp. lite mayonnaise
- 2 white Panini buns
- 1 cup eggplant, sliced
- 1 red or green peppers sliced
- 1/2 zucchini sliced
- 1/4 cup of roasted onion
- 1/2 tbsp. pesto sauce
- 1 cup thinly sliced cooked roast beef

Directions:

1. First, preheat the oven to 450 F.
2. Then, place eggplant, red or green peppers, zucchini over a baking tray lined with parchment paper; put the baking tray in the oven for 10 minutes until the veggies are tender.

3. Remove from the oven and seal with foil; let it rest for 15 minutes.
4. Slice buns in half and set aside.
5. Mix pesto sauce with mayonnaise. Spread on the inside of each bun.
6. Set each with 1/2 cup of sliced roast beef and roasted vegetables.

Nutrition Facts Per Serving:

Calories: 356.93 kcal
Protein 20.17 g
Carbohydrates 36.77 g
Total Fat: 14.56g
Sodium: 931.63 mg
Potassium: 860 mg
Phosphorus: 200 mg

107. Chicken Sandwich (Healthy, Low Caloric)

Preparation time: 10 minutes

Cooking time: 20 minutes

Servings: 1

Ingredients:

- 1 piece Boston leaf lettuce
- 1.8 oz. chicken breast, grilled and cooled
- 1/2 green onion, sliced
- 1/4 cup seedless grapes, halved
- 1/2 tbsp. low-fat mayonnaise
- 1/4 cup celery, diced
- 1/8 tsp. cinnamon
- 1/2 tbsp. lemon juice
- 1/2 cup of fresh basil leaves
- 2 slices white bread, toasted

Directions:

1. Mix all ingredients, except lettuce, basil, and bread, in a large bowl.
2. Then, spread a small amount of the mixture over toast and top with basil.
3. Place Boston lettuce leaf on top, cover with the second toast and serve.

Nutrition Facts Per Serving:

Calories: 34.02 kcal
Protein 2.12 g
Carbohydrates: 5.39 g
Total Fat: 0.65 g
Sodium: 46.74 mg
Potassium: 130 mg
Phosphorus: 28 mg

108. Tomato Stuffed Portobello Caps (Healthy, Low Caloric)

Preparation time: 6 minutes

Cooking time: 11 minutes

Servings: 2

Ingredients:

- 2/3 cup tomatoes, chopped
- 1/2 cup mozzarella cheese, shredded
- 2 tsp. extra virgin olive oil
- 1 tsp. minced garlic
- 1/8 tsp. ground pepper
- 1/2 tsp. rosemary, finely chopped
- 2 tbsp. lemon juice
- 2 tsp. low sodium soy sauce
- 4 Portobello mushroom caps

Directions:

1. Take a bowl and mix tomatoes, 1 teaspoon

olive oil, garlic and pepper.

2. Preheat the grill to medium heat.
3. In a small bowl, merge 1 teaspoon olive oil, soy sauce, and lemon juice.
4. Discard the stem from the mushrooms and garnish the insides of the mushroom caps with the oil mixture.
5. Grill the mushroom caps stem sides down and let it cook for five minutes on each side.
6. Detach from the grill and fill with the tomato filling.
7. Top with mozzarella cheese. Return the mushroom to the grill and cook until the cheese has melted.

Nutrition Facts Per Serving:

Calories: 146 Kcal
Fat: 3.52 g
Fiber: 6 g
Carbs: 15.76 g
Protein: 17.97 g

Sodium: 440mg
Potassium: 1256mg
Phosphorus: 537mg

109. Swordfish and Citrus Salsa Delight (Healthy, Low Caloric)

Preparation time: 10 minutes

Cooking time: 15 minutes

Servings: 3

Ingredients:

- 1/4 pounds swordfish steaks
- 1/2 tbsp. pineapple juice concentrate (thawed)
- 1/8 tsp. cayenne pepper
- 1/2 tbsp. olive oil
- 1/4 cup fresh orange juice
- 1/2 tbsp. chopped fresh cilantro
- 1 tsp. white sugar
- 1/2 tbsp. diced red bell pepper
- 1 1/2 tbsp. orange juice
- 1 jalapeno peppers (seeded and minced)

141

- 1/8 cup diced fresh mango
- 1/4 cup canned pineapple chunks (undrained)
- 1/2 orange (peeled, and cut into bite-size)

Directions:

1. In a bowl, make the salsa by combining and mixing well orange, cilantro, sugar, mango, pineapple chunks, diced red bell pepper, minced jalapenos, and 1 1/2 tablespoons orange juice. Then, cover the bowl and refrigerate.
2. Take a non-reactive bowl and mix the pineapple juice concentrate, cayenne pepper, olive oil, and 1/4 cup orange juice.
3. Add swordfish steaks in the bowl of pineapple juice mixture. Coat and turn well.
4. Ensure to marinate for about 30 minutes.
5. On a gas grill, set heat to medium-high. For 12 to 15 minutes in total, grill the swordfish on both sides, then serve with salsa.

Nutrition Facts Per Serving:

Calories: 348.54
Total Fat: 13.65 g
Fiber: 16 g
Carbs: 4.45 g
Protein: 23.51 g
Sugars: 3.82 g
Sodium: 107.79 mg
Potassium: 456.7 mg
Phosphorus: 34.5 mg

110. Basic Meatloaf

Preparation Time: 5 minutes
Cooking time: 45 minutes
Servings: 8

Ingredients:

- 0.5 pound lean ground turkey
- 1 egg white
- 1 tablespoon lemon juice
- 1/2 cup plain breadcrumbs

- 1/2 teaspoon onion powder
- 1/2 teaspoon Italian seasoning
- 1/4 teaspoon black pepper
- 1/2 cup chopped onions
- 1/2 cup diced green bell pepper
- 1/4 cup of water

Directions:

1. Mix the meat with the lemon juice thoroughly in a bowl.
2. Stir in the remaining seasoning, breadcrumbs, egg white, veggies, and water.
3. Mix well, and then spread this mixture in a loaf pan.
4. Bake the crumbly meatloaf for 45 minutes at 350 degrees F.
5. Slice and serve.

Nutrition Facts Per Serving:

Calories: 632.71 kcal
Total Fat: 31.14 g
Carbs: 40.94 g

Protein: 47.15 g
Sodium: 501.63 mg
Potassium: 711 mg
Phosphorus 500 mg

111. Feta and Spinach Pita Bake

Preparation Time: 10 minutes

Cooking Time: 20 Minutes

Servings: 6

Ingredients:

- 2 Roma tomatoes, chopped
- 6 Whole wheat Pita bread
- 1 Jar sun dried tomato pesto
- 4 Mushrooms, fresh and sliced
- 1 Bunch spinach, rinsed and chopped
- 2 Tablespoons cheddar cheese, grated
- 3 Tablespoons olive oil
- 1/2 Cup of Feta cheese, crumbled
- Dash black pepper

143

Directions:

1. Start by heating the oven to 350, and get to your pita bread. Spread the tomato pesto on the side of each one. Put them in a baking pan with the tomato side up.
2. Top with tomatoes, spinach, mushrooms, cheddar, and feta. Splash with olive oil and season with pepper.
3. Bake for twelve minutes, and then serve cut into quarters.

Nutrition Facts Per Serving:

Calories: 700.42 kcal
Total Fat: 55.34 g
Carbs: 48.3 g
Sugars: 8.33 g
Protein: 19.98 g
Sodium: 1107.21 mg
Potassium: 1000 mg
Phosphorus: 300 mg

112. Roasted Halibut with Banana-orange Relish

Preparation time: 10 minutes

Cooking time: 10 minutes

Servings: 2

Ingredients:

- 1/4 cup cilantro
- 1/2 tsp. freshly grated orange zest
- 1/2 tsp. kosher salt, divided
- 1 lb. halibut or any deep-water fish
- 1 tsp. ground coriander, divided into half
- 2 oranges (peeled, segmented and chopped)
- 2 ripe bananas, diced
- 2 tbsp. lime juice

Directions:

1. First, preheat the oven at 450 F.
2. In a pan, prepare the fish by rubbing 1/2 tsp.

coriander and 1/4 tsp. kosher salt.

3. Place in a baking sheet with cooking spray and bake for 10 minutes.
4. Then, stir the orange zest, bananas, chopped oranges, lime juice, cilantro and the rest of the salt and coriander in a medium bowl, to prepare the relish.
5. Spoon the relish over the roasted fish.

Nutrition Facts Per Serving:

Calories: 337 kcal

Fat: 5 g

Fiber: 6 g

Carbs: 46.01 g

Protein: 30.82 g

Sodium: 1257 mg

Potassium: 1049 mg

Phosphorus: 633 mg

113. Salad Greens with Roasted Beets (Low Caloric)

Preparation time: 10 minutes

Cooking time: 60 minutes

Servings: 2

Ingredients:

- 1/8 cup extra-virgin olive oil
- 1/4 cup chopped walnuts
- 1/4 teaspoon Dijon mustard
- 1/2 tablespoon dried cranberries, chopped roughly
- 1/2 tablespoon minced red onions
- 1 tablespoon sherry vinegar
- 1 1/2 medium beets, washed and trimmed
- 2 cups baby spinach

Directions:

1. Take an aluminum foil and wrap beets. Then,

bake in a preheated oven at 400 F, for about 1 hour.

2. Once done, open foil and allow cooling.
3. When cool to touch, peel beets and dice.
4. Take a large bowl and mix well mustard, red onions, vinegar, and olive oil. Mix in spinach, beets and cranberries. Toss to coat well.

Nutrition Facts Per Serving:

Calories: 156 kcal
Fat: 12.57 g
Fiber: 3.1 g
Carbs: 9.21 g
Protein: 3.48 g
Sodium: 195 mg
Potassium: 426 mg
Phosphorus: 78 mg

114. Maple Glazed Steak

Preparation time: 6 minutes + 4 hours marinating

Cooking time: 10 minutes

Servings: 4

Ingredients:

- 0.5 lbs. flank steak
- 1/4 teaspoon salt-free meat tenderizer powder
- 1/4 teaspoon stevia
- 2 tablespoons lemon juice
- 2 tablespoons low sodium soy sauce
- 1 tablespoon maple syrup

Directions:

1. Pound the meat with a mallet then place it in a shallow dish.
2. Drizzle the meat tenderizer powder over the meat.
3. Whisk the rest of the ingredients and spread this marinade over the meat.

4. Marinate the meat for 4 hours in the refrigerator.
5. Bake the meat for 5 minutes per side at 350 degrees F.
6. Slice and serve.

Nutrition Facts Per Serving:

Calories: 571 kcal
Total Fat: 18.9 g
Cholesterol: 125 mg
Sodium: 385 mg
Carbohydrates: 2.1 g
Protein: 99 g
Calcium: 36 mg
Phosphorous: 930 mg
Potassium: 2004 mg

115. Herb Crusted Roast Leg of Lamb

Preparation time: 15 minutes

Cooking time: 60 minutes

Servings: 12

Ingredients:

- 1 or(4 lb.). leg of lamb
- 3 tsp. lemon juice
- 2 minced cloves garlic
- 1 tbsp. curry powder
- 1/2 tsp. ground black pepper
- 1/2 cup vermouth, dry
- 1 cup sliced onions

Directions:

1. Preheat the oven to 400° F.
2. In a roasting pan, place the lamb's leg. Sprinkle with 1 tsp. lemon juice.
3. Use 2 tsp. of lemon juice and the remaining spices to make the mixture. Rub the mixture into the lamb.
4. Roast the lamb for 30 minutes in the oven at 400° F.
5. Drain the fat and add vermouth and the onions.
6. Now reduce the heat to 325° F and simmer for an extra 1/2 hour.
7. Leave to rest for 3 minutes at least before serving.

Calories: 680 kcal

Protein: 56.35 g

Total Fat: 43.79 g

Carbs: 6.44 g

Sodium: 179.84 mg

Phosphorus: 540 mg

Potassium: 856.25 mg

116. Herb-Crusted Pork Loin (Healthy)

Preparation time: 15 minutes

Cooking time: 40 minutes

Servings: 14

Ingredients:

- 2 tbsp. low sodium soy sauce
- 1 pork loin roast, boneless; about 1 pound
- 2 tbsp. fennel seed
- 2 tbsp. anise seed
- 2 tbsp. dill seed
- 2 tbsp. caraway seed

Directions:

1. Apply soy sauce over the roast until all over is coated. Stir together the fennel, anise seed, dill seed, and caraway in a 13' x 10' x 1' baking pan. Roll pork roast in seeds to coat equally and wrap the meat in a foil; put it in the fridge for 2 hours or overnight.
2. Set the oven to 325°F and remove the foil. In a shallow open roasting pan, put the meat fat side up on the rack.
3. Insert the meat thermometer such that the tip is in the middle of the thickest section.
4. Now Roast pork loin for 35-40 minutes in the baking pan.
5. When roast is done, the meat thermometer should record 145 ° F. Let it rest for 3 minutes. Slice and serve.

Calories: 430 kcal

Protein: 24 g

Sodium: 134 mg

Phosphorus: 225 mg

Dietary Fiber: 1.0 g

Potassium: 405 mg

117. Black Bean Burger and Cilantro Slaw (Healthy, Low Caloric)

Preparation time: 15 minutes

Cooking time: 14 minutes

Servings: 3

Ingredients:

- 1/2 cup bulgur wheat (to prepare mix 1/2 cup bulgur wheat with 1/2 cup hot water and set aside for at least 30 minutes)
- 1/2 cup low sodium, drained, rinsed, mashed, and dried black beans
- 1 tsp. ground black pepper
- 1/2 tsp. smoked paprika
- 1 tsp. granulated garlic
- 1 tsp. onion flakes
- 1 tbsp. Reduced sodium, French's Worcestershire sauce
- 1 tbsp. reduced-sodium, Better Than Bouillon beef
- 1/2 cup scallions
- 1/2 cup onions (sautéed until translucent)
- 3 hamburger rolls
- 2 tbsp. sesame oil
- 2 tbsp. cilantro
- 1/4 cup lime juice
- 1/4 cup balsamic vinegar
- 1/4 cup lite mayonnaise
- 3 cups slaw mix, 10-oz. bag
- 2 tbsp. flour
- 2 tbsp. canola oil for searing
- zest of one lime

Directions:

1. Preheat the oven to 400° F.
2. Combine onion flakes, granulated garlic, beef

149

bouillon, ground black pepper, Worcestershire sauce, black beans, smoked paprika, bulgur wheat, half a cup of scallions and onions in a medium-sized bowl.

3. Now mold half a cup of the mixture into the burgers and refrigerate (or freeze) until firmly formed (not frozen).

4. Make vinaigrette by combining 1 tbsp. of cilantro, lime juice, sesame oil, and vinegar together.

5. In a small bowl add all but 2 tbsp. of vinaigrette to the slaw mix and whisk gently, then put aside in the fridge.

6. Add the remaining 2 tbsp. of vinaigrette and the mayonnaise to another small bowl and set aside.

7. Dust the flour on the black bean burgers and remove the excess, then put on the pre-sprayed pan and also spray the burger tops. Bake for at least 14 minutes and flip around burgers halfway through.

8. Toast rolls and adds an equal quantity of mayonnaise. Add the black bean burger and cover with around 1/4 cup (or the quantity you want) of slaw.

9. Optional: Gently grill, on medium-high, the black bean burger with the canola oil on either side for about 3-4 minutes if you are in a rush.

Nutrition Facts Per Serving:

Calories: 909.97 kcal
Total Fat: 33.8 g
Carbs: 21.5 g
Protein: 30.82 g
Sodium: 800.21 mg
Phosphorus: 320 mg
Dietary Fiber: 5 g
Potassium: 1100.08 mg

118. Egg, Bacon, and Shrimp Grit Cakes with Cheese Sauce

Note: this is a complete dish. Eat it without side.

> **Preparation time: 15 minutes**
> **Cooking time: 45 minutes**
> **Servings: 6**

Ingredients:

- 2 beaten eggs
- 1/2 cup chicken stock (no added salt)
- 1/4 cup chopped chives
- 4 slices bacon, cubed in 1/2-inch pieces, reduced-sodium
- 1/2 cup diced onions
- 1 tsp. Old Bay Seasoning, low sodium
- 12 16/20 count, chopped, peeled, raw, and deveined shrimp
- 1/2 tsp. ground black pepper
- 1/4 cup sharp, shredded cheddar cheese
- 2 tsp. reduced-sodium, Better Than Bouillon chicken flavor
- 2 tbsp. canola oil
- 1/2 cup grits
- 1/2 tsp. smoked paprika
- 2 tbsp. unsalted butter
- 1/4 cup cream, swiss, mozzarella, or feta cheese
- 1 cup milk (1/2 cup for sauce and 1/2 cup of grits)
- 1 tbsp. flour

Directions:

1. In a broad nonstick sauté pan, scramble the eggs until slightly cooked., then put them in a medium-sized bowl, set aside.
2. Add the butter to the pan and sauté the shrimp, half of the chives, bacon, onions, and Old Bay until the shrimp is slightly pink. Place them in the same bowl as the eggs.
3. Add chicken stock, milk, grits and bouillon using

151

the same pan and cook till done as per package instructions.

4. Turn the heat off and fold the mixture of shrimp, bacon, and egg into grits in the pan. Set the mixture into a 9" x 9" baking pan that is lightly oiled and spread until even; after that, cover and refrigerate till firm.

5. Remove and slice into 6 squares. Heat the milk (for sauce) in a saucepan until warm, and whisk in the black pepper, cheese, paprika and the remaining chives until they are melted. Place aside the sauce.

6. Warm up 1/2 of the canola oil in a wide sauté pan. Dust the grit cakes gently with flour and sauté until they are golden brown. Plate over the top with similar quantities of smoky cheese sauce.

Nutrition Facts Per Serving:

Calories: 1043.05 kcal
Total Fat:84.93 g
Carbs: 38.5 g
Protein: 33.57 g
Sodium: 1289.08 mg
Potassium: 637.44 mg
Phosphorus: 520 mg

119. Cranberry Pork Roast

Note: To make this recipe, a Slow Cooker is needed; alternatively, a Dutch oven or any heavy-duty pot with a good lid will work.

Preparation time: 15 minutes
Cooking time: 8-10 hours
Servings: 12

Ingredients:

- 2 lb. pork roast, center-cut
- 1/2 tsp. salt
- 1 tsp. black pepper
- Half cup chopped cranberries
- 1/8 tsp. nutmeg

- 1/8 tsp. ground cloves
- 1/4 cup honey
- 1 tbsp. brown sugar
- 1 tsp. orange peel (zest), grated

Directions

1. Sprinkle the pork roast with salt and pepper. Put it in a slow cooker or a crock-pot.
2. Attach the rest of the ingredients and pour over the roast.
3. Cover and simmer for 8-10 hours on low.
4. From the slow cooker or crock-pot, cut the roast and slice it into 24 pieces., then cover it with a spoonful of drippings.

Nutrition Facts Per Serving:

Calories: 650 kcal
Protein: 80 g
Sodium: 190 mg
Phosphorus: 900 mg
Dietary Fiber: 0.4 g
Potassium: 406 mg

120. Bavarian Pot Roast

Note: To make this recipe, a Slow Cooker is needed; alternatively, a Dutch oven or any heavy-duty pot with a good lid will work.

Preparation time: 15 minutes

Cooking time: 6 or 12 hours depending on temperature

Servings: 12

Ingredients:

- 4 tbsp. water
- 3 lb. beef chuck roast
- 4 tbsp. flour
- 1/2 tsp. pepper
- 1/2 tsp. ground fresh ginger
- 2 cups sliced apples
- 1/2 cup water or apple juice
- 1/2 cup sliced onions
- 3 whole cloves
- 1 tsp. vegetable oil
- Optional garnish: apple slices, fresh

Directions

1. Trim the extra fat off the beef roast then rinse and dry. Apply oil on the roast's top, and sprinkle with ginger and the pepper and, and then apply the entire cloves to the roast. After that, sear the pot roast on both sides in a hot pan with oil.
2. In a slow cooker or crock-pot, put the onions and apples. Add the pot roast and spill juice of apple over the whole roast.
3. Cover and cook for 10-12 hours on low, or at least 5-6 hours on high.
4. Now, take the roast off the slow cooker. Put it aside, keep it warm through.
5. Strain the juices from the pot roast and drain them back into the slow cooker. To lessen the liquid and thicken it, turn the heat to high.
6. Create a smooth paste using flour and water; after that, add it to the slow cooker, mixing while you combine.
7. Cover and simmer until it thickens. Just before serving, spill over the roast.
8. Optional: Garnish with slices of fresh apples.

Nutrition Facts Per Serving:

Calories: 928.54 kcal
Total Fat: 64.82 g
Carbs: 16.91 g
Protein: 66.46 g
Sodium: 222.15 mg
Phosphorus: 600 mg
Dietary Fiber: 1 g
Potassium: 1103.82 mg

121.   Spicy Beef Stir-Fry (Healthy, Low Caloric)

Preparation time: 15 minutes + 20 minutes marinating
Cooking time: 40 minutes
Servings: 4

Ingredients:

- 8 oz. Sliced beef round tip
- 1 large beaten egg
- 1 sliced, green bell pepper
- 2 tbsp. separated corn-starch
- 2 tbsp. water, separated
- 1/2 tsp. sugar
- 3 tbsp. canola oil, separated
- 1/4 tsp. sesame oil
- 1/4 tsp. red chili pepper, ground
- 1 cup sliced onions
- 2 tsp. reduced-sodium, soy sauce
- 1 tbsp. sherry
- Optional garnish: parsley

Directions:

1. Whisk 1 big egg, 1 tbsp. of water, 1 tbsp. of corn-starch, and 1 tbsp. of canola oil in a large bowl and add the beef. For 20 minutes, marinate.
2. Combine the remaining corn-starch and water in a separate bowl and after that, put it aside.
3. In a skillet, heat the rest of the 2 tbsp. of canola oil and add the mixture of meat to it. Cook till the browning of the meat begins.
4. Add the onion, green bell peppers, and chili pepper. Add the sherry and stir fry for a minute. Add sesame oil, soy sauce, and sugar.
5. Thicken with a mixture of corn-starch and water.
6. Optional: Garnish the beef stir-fry with the parsley.

Calories: 350 kcal

Protein: 21 g

Sodium: 169 mg

Phosphorus: 167 mg

Dietary Fiber: 1.5 g

Potassium: 313 mg

122. Healthy, Zesty Orange Tilapia

Preparation time: 15 minutes

Cooking time: 15 minutes

Servings: 4

Ingredients:

- 8 oz. tilapia
- 1/2 cup sliced, green onions
- 1 tsp. ground black pepper
- 1 cup julienned carrots
- 2 tsp. orange peel (zest), grated
- 3/4 cup julienned celery
- 4 tsp. orange juice

Directions:

1. Preheat the oven to 450° F.
2. In a small bowl, mix the orange zest, celery, carrots, and green onions.
3. Cut 4 equal parts of the tilapia. Tear off 4 wide foil squares and brush the foil with a nonstick spray.
4. Place 1/4 of the vegetables slightly off-center on each sheet of the foil and top with fish.
5. Set the top of each one with 1 tsp. of orange juice. Use ground black pepper to season.
6. To make a pouch or an envelope, fold the foil over it, crimp its edges and place the packets of foil on a baking sheet. Bake for roughly 12 minutes (if the fish is thick, 3-5 minutes longer). When done, fish should conveniently split with a fork.
7. Remove and put the pouches directly on the

plates. When opening, be cautious because of the steam.

Nutrition Facts Per Serving:

Calories: 450 kcal
Protein: 24 g
Sodium: 97 mg
Phosphorus: 214 mg
Dietary Fiber: 1.7 g
Potassium: 543 mg

123. Mashed Carrots and Ginger (Low-calorie Snack)

Preparation time: 15 minutes
Cooking time: 32 minutes
Servings: 3

Ingredients:

- 2 cups baby carrots
- 1/2 tsp. fresh chopped ginger
- 1/2 tsp. honey
- 1/2 tsp. Vanilla extract
- 1/2 tsp. black pepper
- Optional garnish: 1 tbsp. chopped fresh chives

Directions

1. At high heat, steam or boil carrots till the carrots are quite tender.
2. Drop heat to low and use a potato masher to mash carrots.
3. Add the remaining ingredients (pepper, vanilla extract, ginger, and honey) and stir till well combined.
4. Optional: Garnish with diced chives and serve.

Nutrition Facts Per Serving:

Calories: 112 Kcal
Protein: 0.1 g
Sodium: 18 mg
Phosphorus: 6 mg
Dietary Fiber: 2 g
Potassium: 60 mg

124. Aromatic Herbed Rice

Preparation time: 15 minutes

Cooking time: 32 minutes

Servings: 6

Ingredients:

- 3 cups rice, cooked (but do not overcook)
- 1/2 tsp. red pepper flakes
- 2 tbsp. chopped fresh oregano
- 2 tbsp. olive oil
- 2 tbsp. chopped fresh cilantro
- 4–5 sliced thin, cloves fresh garlic
- 2 tbsp. chopped fresh chives
- 1 tsp. red wine vinegar

Directions:

1. Set the olive oil in a large skillet over medium-high heat and sauté the garlic lightly.
2. Add rice, herbs, and flakes of red pepper and continue cooking for 2-4 minutes or till well-mixed.
3. Turn off the flame, mix well and add vinegar.
4. Serve

Nutrition Facts Per Serving:

Calories: 134 kcal
Protein: 2 g
Sodium: 6 mg
Phosphorus: 15 mg
Dietary Fiber: 1.8 g
Potassium: 56 mg

125. Sautéed Collard Greens (Healthy, Low Caloric)

Preparation time: 15 minutes

Cooking time: 15 minutes

Servings: 6

Ingredients:

- 8 cups fresh, blanched, and chopped collard greens
- 2 tbsp. olive oil

- 1 tsp. crushed red pepper flakes
- 1 tbsp. unsalted butter
- 1/4 cup finely diced onions
- 1 tsp. ground black pepper
- 1 tbsp. chopped fresh garlic
- 1 tbsp. vinegar (optional)

Directions:

1. Place the collard greens for 30 seconds in a pot of hot water.
2. Strain off the boiling water and move the greens to a big bowl of ice water quickly. Let the greens cool off, then strain and dry and put them aside.
3. Dissolve the butter and oil together in a wide sauté pan over medium-high flame. Add the onions and garlic and simmer for around 4-6 minutes, until lightly browned. Then add the collard greens and the red and black pepper, and then simmer on high heat for 5-8 minutes, stirring continuously.
4. Remove from the heat and, if needed, add vinegar, and stir.

Nutrition Facts Per Serving:

Calories: 279 kcal
Protein: 2 g
Sodium: 9 mg
Phosphorus: 18 mg
Dietary Fiber: 2.2 g
Potassium: 129 mg

126. Tex Mex Bowl (Healthy)

Preparation time: 15 minutes

Cooking time: 35 minutes

Servings: 4 (bowls)

Ingredients:

- 2 cups canned black beans, low sodium
- 4 tbsp. fresh green onion tops

159

- 2 cups cooked white quinoa, with 1 tsp. of olive oil
- 1/2 cup of salsa
- 2 cups shredded iceberg lettuce
- 40 tortilla corn chips, unsalted
- 1/2 cup regular, cultured sour cream
- 1 cup regular, shredded cheddar cheese

Directions

1. Rinse, drain, and heat the black beans. Take 4 bowls.
2. Into each bowl, layer half a cup of cooked quinoa.
3. To each bowl, add half a cup of black beans.
4. To each bowl, add half a cup of lettuce.
5. Top 2 tbsp. of salsa, 1/4 cup of cheese, 2 tbsp. of sour cream, and 1 tbsp. of green onions to each bowl.
6. Serve each bowl with ten tortilla chips.

Nutrition Facts Per Serving:

Calories: 498 kcal

Protein: 21 g

Sodium: 599 mg

Phosphorus: 472 mg

Dietary Fiber: 13 g

Potassium: 681 mg

127. Pasta with a Cheesy Meat Sauce

Preparation time: 15 minutes

Cooking time: 35 minutes

Servings: 6

Ingredients:

- 1 lb. ground beef
- 1/2 box pasta noodles
- 1 tbsp. onion flakes
- 3/4 cup shredded pepper jack
- 1/2 cup diced onions
- 1 tbsp. Better Than Bouillon beef (no salt added)
- 11/2 cups reduced or no sodium beef stock

160

- 8 oz. softened cream cheese
- 1 tbsp. tomato sauce (no salt added)
- 1/2 tsp. Italian seasoning
- 1/2 tsp. ground black pepper
- 2 tbsp. Reduced sodium, French's Worcestershire sauce

Directions:

1. Cook pasta noodles.
2. Cook the ground beef, onions, and onion flakes in a large skillet till the meat is browned.
3. Rinse and add bouillon, stock, and tomato sauce.
4. Bring to a boil, occasionally stirring. Blend in the cooked pasta, turn off the heat and add the cream cheese, seasonings (Worcestershire sauce, black pepper, and Italian seasoning) and shredded cheese. Stir in the pasta mixture till all the cheese is melted.

Nutrition Facts Per Serving:

Calories: 502 kcal
Protein: 23 g
Sodium: 401 mg
Phosphorus: 278 mg
Dietary Fiber: 1.7 g
Potassium: 549 mg

128. Rice Pilaf Baked in Pumpkin

Preparation time: 15 minutes
Cooking time: 60 minutes
Servings: 8

Ingredients:

- 2 cups cooked rice (made without salt)
- Fresh herbs of your desire (cilantro, parsley, basil), black pepper or dried herbs
- 1 raw pumpkin (1 lb.)
- 2 stalks diced celery (or customize with zucchini, peppers, vegetables, or okra)
- 2 small, diced onions

- 2 diced and peeled carrots
- 2 chopped cloves garlic
- 2 tbsp. canola oil
- 0.5 cup cranberries, dried or fresh

Directions:

1. Both the rice pilaf and pumpkin shell can be cooked ahead of time and kept separately in the fridge till it's time to place it in the oven.
2. Cut the top of the pumpkin carefully to make the pumpkin shell. When put back on the pumpkin, just make sure it would fit snugly. Set it aside.
3. To make the shell empty, clean the inside of the pumpkin. Discard all the seeds and the material inside.
4. Place the pumpkin on a baking pan or a cookie sheet lined with foil. (Store the pumpkin in the fridge if making ahead.)

Preparation for Filling:

1. If not already prepared, prepare the rice to make the pilaf filling. Put it aside.
2. In a saucepan, sauté all the vegetables (celery, onions, garlic, carrots) in canola oil till they are tendered.
3. Stir in the cranberries, seasonings, and rice.

To Bake:

1. Preheat the oven to 350F.
2. Spoon the rice pilaf gently into the hollow pumpkin shell and replace the pumpkin top to cover. Put it in a casserole dish if you're not using a pumpkin.
3. Bake for almost 60 minutes or till a fork or knife easily pierces the pumpkin shell. Cover and bake for just 30 minutes or till completely cooked when using a casserole dish.
4. Let it cool for 15 minutes at least.

5. Serve it warm or at room temperature with a large serving spoon by pulling servings out of the shell.

6. To make 8 to 12 wedges, slice through the pumpkin for more fun. Serve the wedge with the pilaf. It'll make the pumpkin tender but firm. Eat just the pumpkin flesh and remove the tough skin.

Nutrition Facts Per Serving:

Calories: 760 kcal
Protein: 5 g
Sodium: 40 mg
Phosphorus: 110 mg
Potassium: 426 mg

129. BBQ Ribs with Marinade

Preparation time: 15 minutes
Cooking time: 35 minutes
Servings: 16

Ingredients:

- 2 tbsp. brown sugar
- ½ lb. beef ribs
- 1/4 cup honey
- 2 tbsp. finely chopped, sweet onion
- 1/4 cup apple cider vinegar
- 1 grated or chopped garlic clove
- 1 cup of water
- 2 tbsp. tomato paste
- 2 tsp. dry mustard
- 1 tbsp. all-purpose flour
- 1 tsp. brown seasoning sauce
- 1 tsp. hot pepper sauce
- 1/4 tsp. Salt
- 1-1/2 tbsp. butter, unsalted

Directions:

BBQ Marinade for the Ribs:

1. Have the onions finely diced and the garlic clove minced.

2. Dissolve the butter in a saucepan over a low flame.

3. Add the garlic and onion and heat till slightly browned.

4. Except for the flour, add the rest of the ingredients.
5. Continue to heat and stir until mixed, and the sauce continues to simmer lightly over medium flame. Reduce the flame and add flour.
6. Whisk till it is mixed and the sauce continues to thicken. Cover the saucepan and set aside for the BBQ grill to marinate the ribs.
7. Set it frozen until you are ready to thaw or use or refrigerate for about 7 days if not used immediately.

Prep Instructions:

8. Remove the ribs rack from the package. (Scrape off the skin on the back of the rack only if the butcher hasn't already done so.)
9. Place the ribs rack, with the bottom side up, on the foil.
10. Add the marinade to the bottom of the rack, and then turn it over.
11. Apply some marinade to the rack's top and turn the foil over, covering the top and sides cautiously so that no marinade spills out.
12. Save some leftover marinade for the last caramelizing phase on the grill or some for dipping while eating.
13. Put your foil coated ribs into the fridge to marinate as you prepare the grill.

Nutrition Facts Per Serving:

Calories: 369.58 kcal
Total Fat: 18.68g
Carbs: 35.41g
Protein: 15.96 g
Sodium: 285.79 mg
Phosphorus: 163 mg
Potassium: 400.88 mg

130. Shrimp and Coconut Curry Noodle Bowl

Preparation time: 15 minutes

Cooking time: 20 minutes

Servings: 5

Ingredients:

- 2 tbsp. coconut oil
- 4 oz. rice noodles
- 2 diced summer squash or zucchini
- 1 diced sweet onion
- 2 grated or minced cloves garlic
- 2 corn kernels, ears sweet
- 2-3 tbsp. Thai red curry paste
- 1 tbsp. grated fresh ginger
- 1/3 or 1/2 cup water
- 4-oz. full fat, can coconut milk
- 2 tsp. honey
- 1 tbsp. soy sauce, low sodium
- Top with 1/4 cup cilantro, fresh (or roughly chopped basil)
- Zest and juice from half a lime

Directions:

1. Cook the rice noodles by water.
2. In a broad skillet, heat the coconut oil. Add in onion and cook over a high flame for at least 5 minutes. Add the corn, zucchini, ginger, and garlic and cook for 5 more minutes till it begins to get soft.
3. Mix in the curry paste and simmer for another minute.
4. Stir in the water, coconut milk, honey, and soy sauce. Bring it to boil, and simmer till the mixture starts to thicken (about 5 minutes). You may add a little water if the sauce gets too thick.
5. Remove the skillet from the flame. Add either the basil or cilantro, according to preference, then whisk in the zest and lime juice.

6. Distribute the rice noodles into different bowls for serving and top with a mixture of curry.

Nutrition Facts Per Serving:

Calories: 418 kcal
Protein: 16 g
Sodium: 195 mg
Phosphorus: 285 mg
Dietary Fiber: 5 g
Potassium: 660 mg

131. Curried Turkey with Rice

Preparation time: 15 minutes
Cooking time: 25 minutes
Servings: 6

Ingredients:

- 0.5 lb. turkey breast, sliced into eight cutlets (2 oz.)
- 1 tsp. vegetable oil
- 1 tbsp. margarine, unsalted
- 1 cup white rice, cooked
- 1 chopped, medium onion
- 2 tbsp. flour
- 1 cup chicken broth, low-sodium
- 2 tsp. curry powder
- 1 tsp. sugar
- 1/2 cup creamer, non-dairy

Directions:

1. In a broad skillet, heat the oil. Add the turkey and cook, flipping once till no longer pink for at least 10 minutes. Put the turkey on a dish. Wrap in a foil to stay warm.
2. In the same skillet, melt the margarine. Add the curry powder and onion. Cook, then attach flour while stirring continuously.
3. Stir in sugar, broth, and non-dairy creamer. Stir often till thickened.
4. Transfer turkey to the skillet. Cook, flipping to coat till heated through, for approximately 2 minutes.
5. Sauce over rice and serve the turkey.

Nutrition Facts Per Serving:

Calories: 450 kcal

Protein: 8 g

Sodium: 27 mg

Phosphorus: 88 mg

Dietary Fiber: 1 g

Potassium: 156 mg

132. Marinated Shrimp

Preparation time: 15 minutes

Cooking time: 25 minutes

Servings: 12

Ingredients:

- 1 1/2 cup oil
- 2.5 lb. large shrimp
- 8 bay leaves
- 2 1/2 tsp. undrained capers
- 3/4 cup white vinegar
- 1 tsp. Salt
- 1 1/2 tsp. celery seeds
- 1 pared, minced garlic clove
- 1 tsp. whole cloves
- 2 cups pared, thinly sliced onions
- Two dashes of sauce or red pepper

Directions:

1. Combine all the ingredients mentioned above to make a mixture.
2. Take two half lb. large shrimp, which is deveined and cooked in a crab boil. Apply the mixture.
3. Alternate the layers of onions, bay leaves, and shrimp mixture in a glass bowl, and place it in a refrigerator for 24 hours. Enjoy.

Nutrition Facts Per Serving:

Calories: 617.61kcal

Total Fat: 57.65g

Carbs: 8.32g

Protein: 17.46g

Sodium: 808.22mg

Potassium: 241.46mg

Phosphorus: 30 mg

133. Honey Garlic Chicken (Healthy, Low Caloric)

Preparation time: 15 minutes

Cooking time: 1 hour

Servings: 4

Ingredients:

- 2 lb. roasting chicken
- 1/2 cup honey
- 1 tsp. garlic powder
- 1 tbsp. olive oil
- 1/2 tsp. black pepper

Directions:

1. Preheat the oven to 350° F.
2. Grease olive oil on a baking pan.
3. Put the chicken in the pan and avoid overlapping pieces, then coat the chicken with honey and seasonings.
4. Bake for at least 1 hour or until both the sides are brown. During cooking, turn once.

Nutrition Facts Per Serving:

Calories: 570 kcal
Protein: 13 g
Dietary Fiber: 0 g
Sodium: 40 mg
Phosphorus: 99 mg
Potassium: 144 mg

134. Chili Con Carne with Rice

Preparation time: 15 minutes

Cooking time: 1-½ hours

Servings: 7

Ingredients:

- Half lb. lean ground beef
- 1/2 cup pinto beans, cooked (without salt)
- 1 can (6 oz.) tomato paste, no-salt-added
- 1 cup green pepper, chopped
- 1 tsp. ground cumin
- 2 tsp. garlic powder
- 1 cup onion, chopped
- 1 tsp. paprika
- 3 1/2 cups rice, cooked

- 3 cups of water

Directions:

1. In a big pot, brown the ground beef and extract the fat.
2. Add the onion and green pepper and cook till the onion becomes transparent. Attach the rest of the ingredients and cook for 1-1/2 hours.
3. Serve over scalding hot rice.

Nutrition Facts Per Serving:

Calories: 1119.65 kcal
Total Fat: 24.95 g
Carbs: 152.82 g
Protein: 69.4 g
Sodium: 222.29 mg
Phosphorus: 863.82 mg
Dietary Fiber: 2 g
Potassium: 2677.01 mg

Dessert

135. Pineapple Cream Cake

Preparation time: 15 minutes

Cooking time: 1 hour 15 minutes

Servings: 18

Ingredients:

- 3 eggs
- 1 tsp. vanilla flavoring
- 1/4 cup stevia
- 1 (8 oz.) drained crushed pineapple, canned
- 1 cup water
- 18 oz. yellow cake box mix
- 1/3 cup vegetable oil
- 8 oz. pack softened cream cheese

Directions:

1. Preheat the oven to a suitable temperature on the cake mix box.
2. Combine stevia, cream cheese, and 1 egg in a shallow cup, stirring well. Whisk in, Stir in. The pineapple was drained and put aside.
3. Combine the cake mix, water, oil, vanilla flavoring, and the remaining 2 eggs in a big dish. Beat at fast speed around two minutes using a food processor.
4. Spray with oil spray, Bundt pan, and then dust with flour.
5. Mix well with the cheese mixture in the cake batter. Then mix in the oiled and floured pan with the batter.
6. Bake or until the middle is prepared, about 65 minutes. The doneness measure is achieved by sticking a bread knife in the middle of the cake, for 10 minutes, cool in the container.

Nutrition Facts Per Serving:

Calories: 906.04 kcal
Total Fat: 82.62 g
Fiber: 6 g

Carbs: 49.52 g

Sugars: 45.83 g

Protein: 15.74 g

Sodium: 453.58 mg

Potassium: 380 mg

Phosphorus: 250 mg

136. Sugarless Pecan and Raisin Cookies (Healthy)

Preparation time: 15 minutes

Cooking time: 20 minutes

Servings: 42 (cookies)

Ingredients:

- 2 tsp. baking powder
- 1/2 tsp. grated orange rind
- 1/2 tsp. salt
- 1/2 tsp. cinnamon
- 1 egg
- 3/4 cup unsweetened orange juice, canned
- 1/4 cup oil
- 1/2 cup raisins
- 1/2 cup pecans
- 1 3/4 cup flour

Directions:

1. Mix the baking powder, flour, and cinnamon.
2. The remainder of the ingredients is applied.
3. Mix thoroughly.
4. On an ungreased baking sheet, drop only by the teaspoonful.
5. Bake at 375F for 20 minutes.

Nutrition Facts Per Serving:

Calories: 1017.11 kcal

Total Fat: 50.17 g

Cholesterol: 41 mg

Carbohydrate: 129.01 g

Sugars: 31.82 g

Protein: 18.25 g

Sodium: 1110.34 mg

Phosphorous: 320 mg

Potassium: 700 mg

137. Sugar Cookies

Preparation time: 1 hour

Cooking time: 10 minutes

Servings: 20

Ingredients:

- 1 tbsp. creamer, non-dairy
- 11/2 tsp. baking powder
- 1 cup stevia
- 1/2 cup margarine, unsalted
- 1 tsp. vanilla
- 1/2 tsp. salt
- 1 well-beaten egg
- 2 cups flour, sifted
- 1 tsp. red coloring

Directions:

1. Sieve baking powder, 11/2 cups of flour, and salt together.
2. Creamy margarine; progressively mix cream and stevia until smooth and creamy. Add the vanilla, egg, red coloring, and creamer. Add the filtered dry components, and add the remaining 1/2 cup of flour steadily until the dough is firm enough to tackle. Chill out for 1 hour at least.
3. Roll the mixture 1/8 inch in thickness on a thinly floured board, then shape them and put on floured baking sheets. Add sugar to sprinkle. Bake for 8-10 min in an oven at 375°F.

Nutrition Facts Per Serving:

Calories: 500 kcal

Total Fat: 12.1 g

Cholesterol: 27 mg

Carbohydrate: 4.7 g

Sugars: 0.8 g

Protein: 3.2 g

Phosphorous: 120 mg

Potassium: 100 mg

138. Summer Fruit Cobbler

Preparation time: 15 minutes

Cooking time: 50 minutes

Servings: 6

Ingredients:

- 4 cups blackberries or strawberries
- 1 cup brown granulated sugar
- 1 egg
- 1 cup white flour
- 1/2 tsp. baking powder
- 1/4 cup butter

Directions:

1. The oven should be preheated to 375F. The berries are sliced/cleaned and are cut into tiny pieces. Put them in an 8 by 13 baking dish.
2. Combine together the sugar, baking powder, and flour in a reasonably sized dish.
3. Attach the egg and blend until the mixture is grainy, using a mixer.
4. Then dice the butter at room temperature, and place it in the tub, then blend it until it is fully mixed with the beaters. It's always going to look crumbly.
5. Spread over the berries like this.
6. Bake for about 50 minutes, based on the brownness of the crust you like. Ensure it is bubbling. Slightly cool.

Nutrition Facts Per Serving:

Calories: 660 kcal

Protein: 9 g

Carbohydrates: 40 g

Fat: 2 g

Sodium: 160 mg

Potassium: 580 mg

Phosphorus: 206 mg

139. Berries Napoleon

Preparation time: 15 minutes

Cooking time: 10 minutes

Servings: 6

Ingredients:

- 1 tbsp. powdered brown sugar
- 12 wonton wrappers
- 1/2 cup blueberries
- 2 tbsp. granulated sugar
- 1 cup fat-free Reddi-Wip whipped topping
- 1/2 cup raspberries

Directions:

1. Preheat the oven at 400F.
2. Using a baking sheet that suits 12 wonton wrappers, apply the oil spray.
3. Spread wonton wrappers out and sprinkle cooking spray on them.
4. Sprinkle wonton wrappers with granulated sugar.
5. Bake wontons until golden brown or for 5 minutes; detach from baking sheet.
6. Put on a serving tray with 6 wonton wrappers.
7. With 2 tbsp. whipped topping, 1 tbsp. raspberries and 1 tbsp. blueberries fill each wrapper.
8. Get a 2nd wonton wrapping on top of the berries.
9. By powdered sugar, dust the tops. If needed, pour over a spoonful of whipped cream, berries, and mint leaves. Serve Right away.

Nutrition Facts Per Serving:

Calories: 287 kcal

Fat: 23 g

Carbohydrates: 1 g

Protein: 31 g

Sodium: 280 mg

Potassium: 150 mg

Phosphorus: 75 mg

140. Blueberry Cream Cones

Preparation time: 15 minutes
Cooking time: 6 hours
Servings: 4

Ingredients:

- 4 ice-cream small cones
- 1 cup whipped topping
- 1/4 cup blueberry preserves or jam
- 1 1/4 cup fresh blueberries or fresh
- 2 oz. cream cheese

Directions:

1. Soften the cheese. Put it in a container and beat until fluffy and smooth with a high mixer up to 5 mins.
2. Fold in cream cheese with jam and fruit.
3. Mix jam with cups of whipped topping.
4. Fill the cones, and before ready to eat, freeze overnight or for a period of 6 hours at least.

Nutrition Facts Per Serving:

Calories: 340 kcal
Total Fat: 8.92 g
Carbs: 64.09 g
Sugars: 36.51 g
Protein: 5.17 g
Potassium: 111 mg
Sodium: 186 mg
Phosphorus: 57 mg

141. Red, White, and Blue Pie

Preparation time: 15 minutes
Cooking time: none
Servings: 8

Ingredients:

- 9" crust graham cracker
- 1/2 cup red raspberry, low-sugar preserves
- 1 1/2 cup raspberries, fresh
- 3 cups dairy Reddi-Wip® whipped topping
- 8 oz. low-fat whipped cream cheese
- 1 cup blueberries, fresh

Directions:

1. Beat whipped cheese until fluffy with an immersion blender at medium speed to create the filling up to 5 mins.
2. Wrap whipped topping with a combination of cream cheese.
3. Layer the filling uniformly over the cracker crust's rim.
4. Arrange the blueberries throughout the outer circle of the pie before serving. Layer the raspberries along the pie's inner ring.
5. Complete decorating in the middle with 1 spoonful of whipped cream and on top with a strawberry or raspberry.

Nutrition Facts Per Serving:

Calories: 600 mg
Fat: 10 g
Carbohydrates: 55 g
Protein: 14 g

Sodium: 430 mg
Potassium: 670 mg
Phosphorus: 300 mg

142. Frozen Fruit Delight

Preparation time: 15 minutes

Freezing time: 3 hours

Servings: 4

Ingredients:

- 1 cup strawberries, sliced
- 8 oz. crushed canned pineapple
- 1 tbsp. lemon juice
- 1/3 cup maraschino cherries
- 4 oz. sour cream, reduced-fat
- 3 cups dairy Reddi-Wip® whipped topping
- 1/2 cup stevia
- 1/8 tsp. salt

Directions:

1. Drain the pineapple and chop the cherries.
2. In a moderate cup, put all ingredients, excluding

whipped topping, and mix till it's combined. Fold into the whipped topping.

3. Then put the mixture in a tub of plastic, and then freeze for 3 hours before it is hardened.

Nutrition Facts Per Serving:

Calories: 530.69 kcal
Total Fat: 28.39 g
Carbs: 65.73 g
Sugars: 52.99 g
Protein: 7.94 g
Sodium: 199.66 mg
Potassium: 550 mg
Phosphorus: 155 mg

143. Quick Fruit Sorbet

Preparation time: 15 minutes

Cooking time: none

Servings: 8

Ingredients:

- 1 cup unsweetened frozen raspberries
- 4 pitted plums
- 20 oz. frozen crushed pineapple, juice-packed, canned

Directions:

1. Sufficiently Defrost Pineapple to take out of the can.
2. Put all the fruit in the food processor before pureed and refined.
3. Serve instantly or disperse and freeze in an 8" by 8" container.

Nutrition Facts Per Serving:

Calories: 340.91 kcal
Total Fat: 1.11 g
Carbs: 86.36 g
Sugars: 76 g
Protein: 2.9 g
Sodium: 6.37 mg
Potassium: 590 mg
Phosphorus: 52 mg

144. Strawberry Sorbet

Preparation time: 15 minutes
Cooking time: none
Servings: 4

Ingredients:

- 1 1/4 cup ice
- 1 cup fresh or frozen strawberries
- 1/4 cup water
- 1 tbsp. lemon juice

Directions:

1. Merge all the ingredients in the blender and serve.

Nutrition Facts Per Serving:

Calories: 268 kcal
Total Fat: 19.8 g
Saturated Fat: 7.8 g
Cholesterol: 72 mg
Sodium: 307 mg
Carbohydrates: 7 g
Dietary Fiber: 2.4 g
Sugars: 2.1 g
Protein: 4.6 g
Calcium: 44 mg
Phosphorous: 371 mg
Potassium: 135 mg

145. Tropical Ice Cream Sandwiches

Preparation time: 15 minutes
Cooking time: 6 hours
Servings: 15

Ingredients:

- 8 packs No Calorie Splenda Sweetener
- 1 pack unflavored Knox gelatin
- 1 cup dairy Reddi-Wip whipped topping
- 15 oz. crushed pineapple canned in juice
- 1 1/2 cups protein powder Procel
- 12 squares graham cracker

Directions:

1. Cover a 13" by 9 1/2" baking pan using a plastic wrap that helps both sides of the pan to hang at least 10".

2. Arrange and set aside 12 graham cracker pieces in the pan.
3. Drain the pineapple and put 1/2 cup pineapple juice in reserve.
4. Mix the pulped pineapple, Splenda®, and Procel® in a large mixing tub, so you see no blobs.
5. Fold in a whipped cover, and then put it aside. Boil the 1/2 cup pineapple juice in a shallow saucepan.
6. Connect 1 package of Knox® gelatin that is not flavored. Remove from heat and blend until dissolved. On graham crackers, add the mixture equally.
7. Place plastic wrap over the graham crackers from the edges of the pan.
8. Cover with foil made of aluminum and seal tight. Freeze overnight or for a period of 6 hours. "Cut into fifteen 2-1/2" by 2-1/2" bits until freezing and serve.

Nutrition Facts Per Serving:

Calories: 870.29 kcal
Total Fat: 13.25 g
Carbs: 84.81 g
Sugars: 49.9 g
Protein: 106.61 g
Sodium: 398.87 mg
Potassium: 1000:mg
Phosphorus: 1200 mg

146. Watermelon Ice Cream

Preparation time: 15 minutes

Cooking time: 3 hours

Servings: 4

Ingredients:

- 3 cups cubed watermelon
- 2 medium frozen bananas
- 1 pinch sea salt
- 1/4 tsp. vanilla extract
- 2/3 cup coconut milk
- 1 tbsp. honey

Directions:

1. In a mixer, mix both ingredients and move to vacant ice cube containers.
2. Place them to freeze for 3 hrs. Or until they are frozen.
3. Carry the watermelon back to the processor.
4. Mix until it achieves a smooth texture.
5. Put the blend in a jar and bring it back to the freezer too stiff for approximately 25 minutes or until the texture is needed.
6. Present like ice-cream with toppings needed.

Nutrition Facts Per Serving:

Calories: 235 kcal
Total Fat: 19.5 g
Carbohydrates: 56 g
Dietary Fiber: 6 g
Sugars: 39 g
Protein: 2.8 g
Sodium: 76 mg

Potassium: 880 mg
Phosphorus: 130 mg

147. Late Summer Blackberry Tart

Preparation time: 15 minutes

Cooking time: 1 hour and 25 minutes

Servings: 6

Ingredients:

- 2/3 cup sliced plum
- 1 cup flour, unbleached
- 1 pinch sea salt
- 2 tbsp. regular sugar
- 1 egg
- 7 tbsp. cold butter
- 3 tbsp. cold water
- 2/3 cup blackberries

Directions:

1. Preheat the oven at 375F.
2. Mix 1 tbsp. of sugar in a dish with blackberries and plum slices. Just set aside.
3. To yet another mixing dish, apply the remaining flour, salt, and sugar. Whisk in order to blend.

4. Using the fingers to split the butter till the combination is grainy like little peas.
5. Only before the mixture falls together, apply ice water, 1 tbsp. at one time. You don't want messy wet dough; just use enough to keep the dough intact.
6. For 20 minutes, let the dough settle.
7. On parchment paper placed over a flipside baking dish, spread the dough out. A rustic, rough edge would be the result.
8. In the middle, organize the fruit appealingly.
9. Bring the sides together, securing them by pressing the dough.
10. With 1 tbsp. of water, beat the egg.
11. Brush the egg wash on the tart dough. Sprinkle if needed with extra raw sugar.
12. Bake until thoroughly browned and crispy, around 30-35 minutes.
13. Serve it warm.

Nutrition Facts Per Serving:

Calories: 690 kcal
Fat: 41 g
Carbohydrates: 71 g
Protein: 10 g
Phosphorus: 141 mg
Potassium: 270 mg
Sodium: 98 g

148. Apple Chocolate Pecan Treats

Preparation time: 15 minutes

Cooking time: 1 hour 15 minutes

Servings: 12

Ingredients:

- half cup chopped pecans
- 1 tbsp. coconut oil
- 2 Fuji apples

- 5 oz. dark chocolate chips semi-sweet

Directions:

1. Vertically slice the apples (top to bottom) into 1/2-inch bits, around 6 pieces per fruit.
2. With the point of the paring knife, cut the seeds from the middle (comprising core) bits.
3. Melt the chocolate chips for around 2 minutes in the microwave on strong. Alternatively, cook the chocolate over a double boiler: put the chocolate in a metal bowl and place it over a hot water saucepan until it's molten.
4. Incorporate coconut oil till soft.
5. Using a fork or tongs, dunk apple slices in cocoa.
6. On a parchment-lined baking sheet, put each dipped treat.
7. Sprinkle the sliced pecans with around 1 tablespoon each.
8. Refrigerate for 1 hour or until cooked with cocoa.
9. Serve and appreciate it as a nice treat or nutritious snack at any moment.

Nutrition Facts Per Serving:

Calories: 777.57 kcal
Total Fat: 53.68 g
Carbs: 70.12 g
Sugars: 49.52 g
Protein: 7.2 g
Sodium: 9.01 mg
Potassium: 700 mg
Phosphorus: 280 mg

149. Stone Cobbler

Preparation time: 15 minutes

Cooking time: 60 minutes

Servings: 8

Ingredients:

- 1/4 cup packed sugar, brown
- 5 tbsp. unsalted butter

- 1 tsp. cinnamon
- 1 tsp. baking powder
- 2 cups rolled oats
- 2 tbsp. sugar
- 2 tbsp. freshly squeezed lemon juice
- 1/4 cup buttermilk
- ¼ cup water
- 1 1/2 cup slightly undercooked quinoa
- 2 cups peaches
- 1/4 tsp. grated nutmeg
- 1 tsp. vanilla
- Cooking spray

Directions:

1. Preheat the oven to 350F.
2. Using cooking spray to spray the 9 by 13" baking dish.
3. Put the peaches in a mixing bowl with lemon juice and brown sugar. Place 10 minutes free.
4. In a separate, wide mixing bowl, add the sugar, oats, butter, baking powder, nutmeg, and cinnamon.
5. Function with your hands on the products before they become a grainy mixture.
6. Add vanilla and buttermilk. Combine before a dough emerges from the mixture.
7. Spread the quinoa on the base of the baking container in an even layer.
8. Organize peaches and their juices in the ready dish uniformly over quinoa
9. Over the peaches, scatter the dough. Lightly click down.
10. Bake till the pastry becomes lightly browned, and the fruit is moist and bubbling, for around 30 minutes.
11. Serve it warm.

Nutrition Facts Per Serving:

Calories: 1004.35 kcal
Total Fat: 18.74 g
Carbs: 180.42 g
Sugars: 26.29 g
Protein: 33.78 g
Sodium: 295.18 mg

Potassium: 1400 mg
Phosphorus: 1100 mg

150. Rhubarb Cake

Preparation time: 15 minutes

Cooking time: 60 minutes

Servings: 16

Ingredients:

For cake:

- 4 tbsp. unsalted butter
- 2 stalks rhubarb
- 3/4 cup sugar
- 1 egg
- 1 cup plain, low fat yogurt
- 2 cups white flour
- 1/8 tsp. salt
- 1 tsp. baking soda

Topping:

- 1/3 cup packed brown sugar
- 1 tsp. cinnamon
- 1/2 cup chopped walnuts
- 2 tsp. unsalted butter

Directions:

Cake:

1. Preheat the oven at 350°F. Using cooking spray to spray the 8-inch square or circular baking sheet.
2. In a mixing cup, put the sugar and the butter with an immersion blender beat.
3. Crack the egg in the container. Beat before the egg is added once more.
4. Stir in the yogurt and stir until it's smooth.
5. Split into 1-inch bits of rhubarb.
6. In a sieve, pour the starch, baking soda, and salt and stir them in a bowl softly.
7. In butter mix, combine dry ingredients. Apply the rhubarb to the combination and use a spoon to blend properly.
8. Set aside and add the batter to the baking tray.

Toppings:

1. Put the cinnamon and brown sugar in a little bowl with the nuts.
2. Dissolve the butter over low heat in a shallow saucepan.

3. Place hot butter over the cinnamon, sugar, and nuts into a mixing cup.
4. Using a wooden spoon, blend properly.
5. Pour the almond topping in a baking pan over cake mix, spreading uniformly.
6. Bake until it comes out clean with a toothpick incorporated in the middle.

Nutrition Facts Per Serving:

Calories: 1096.94 kcal
Total Fat: 43.44 g
Carbs: 158.13 g
Sugars: 56.78 g
Protein: 24.4 g
Sodium: 242.74 mg
Potassium: 700 mg
Phosphorus: 400 mg

151. Fudgesicles

Preparation time: 15 minutes

Cooking time: 60 minutes

Servings: 8

Ingredients:

- 1 minced chipotle pepper
- 2 cups whole milk
- 2 tbsp. unsweetened cocoa
- 1/2 cup lite heavy cream
- 1/4 cup brown sugar
- 1 pinch sea salt
- 1 tsp. vanilla
- 6 oz. chopped dark chocolate, semi-sweet

Directions:

1. In a big mixing cup, put the sliced chocolate in it.
2. In a wide skillet over a moderate flame, mix the cream, milk, cocoa, sugar, and vanilla together.
3. Set it to a boil, and then remove it from the flame.
4. Pour a variation of milk over the chocolate. Add some salt and allow the

186

chocolate to rest until it melts.

5. Apply the chipotle pepper and pulse till the blend is creamy in a blender.

6. Put into 8 ice pop molds or paper cups of 3 ounces.

7. If you don't have ice pop molds, insert spoons to the center of paper cups 1 hr. later.

8. Freeze for 4-5 hours roughly.

Nutrition Facts Per Serving:

Calories: 895.27 kcal
Total Fat: 52.98 g
Carbs: 91.53 g
Sugars: 73.79 g
Protein: 16.92 g
Sodium: 213.9 mg
Potassium: 1200 mg
Phosphorus: 500 mg

152. Raspberry Pear Sorbet

Preparation time: 15 minutes

Cooking time: 60 minutes

Servings: 8

Ingredients:

- 1/4 cup stevia
- 1/2 pint fresh raspberries
- 1 large pear halves, canned in juice
- 2 tablespoons + 2 teaspoons lime juice
- 1/2 tablespoon pear liqueur or vodka. (Optional)
- 1/2 cup of water

Directions:

1. For sugar syrup, add 1/2 cup of water and the sugar to a small saucepan and bring to a boil. Stir continuously to dissolve sugar. Reduce heat. Simmer, uncovered, for 3 minutes. Remove from heat. Place it in the refrigerator to cool.

2. For the puree, combine raspberries, pear, lime juice, and pear liqueur. Cover; process for 30 seconds or until smooth. Stir in chilled sugar syrup.
3. Prepare according to ice-cream maker instructions or spread mixture in an 8x8x2-inch baking pan and cover. Freeze for 4 hours or until solid. Set it in the food processor and process for 30 seconds or until smooth. Transfer to a 1-quart freezer container; cover and freeze sorbet 6 to 8 hours or until solid Serve with additional raspberries.

Nutrition Facts Per Serving:

Calories: 145.96 kcal
Total Fat: 0.49 g
Carbs: 36.93 g
Sugars: 29.88 g
Protein: 0.99 g
Sodium: 3.09 mg
Potassium: 134 mg
Phosphorus: 25 mg

153. Dark Chocolate Trifle

Preparation time: 10 minutes

Cooking time: 15 minutes

Servings: 4

Ingredients:

- 1 small plain sponge Swiss roll
- 3 oz. custard powder
- 5 oz. hot water
- 16 oz. canned mandarins
- 3 tablespoons sherry
- 5 oz. double cream
- 2 cubes, dark chocolate, grated

Directions:

1. Whisk the custard powder with water in a bowl until dissolved.
2. In a bowl, mix the custard well until it becomes creamy and let it sit for 15 minutes.
3. Spread the Swiss roll and cut it in 4 squares.
4. Place the Swiss roll in the 4 serving cups.

5. Top the Swiss roll with mandarin, custard, cream, and chocolate.
6. Serve.

Nutrition Facts Per Serving:

Calories: 315 kcal
Total Fat: 13.5 g
Saturated Fat: 8.4 g
Cholesterol: 43 mg
Sodium: 185 mg
Carbohydrates: 40.1 g
Sugars: 9.1 g
Protein: 2.9 g
Phosphorous: 184 mg
Potassium: 129 mg

154. Pineapple Meringues

> **Preparation time: 10 minutes**
> **Cooking time: 0 minutes**
> **Servings: 4**

Ingredients:

- 4 meringue nests
- 8 oz. crème fraîche
- 2 oz. stem ginger, chopped
- 8 oz. can pineapple chunks

Directions:

1. Place the meringue nests on the serving plates.
2. Whisk the ginger with crème Fraiche and pineapple chunks.
3. Divide the pineapple mixture over the meringue nests.
4. Serve.

Nutrition Facts Per Serving:

Calories: 312 kcal
Total Fat: 22.8 g
Saturated Fat: 0 g
Cholesterol: 0 mg
Carbohydrates: 25 g
Sugars: 23.1 g
Protein: 2.3 g
Phosphorous: 104 mg
Potassium: 110 mg

155. Baked Custard

Preparation time: 10 minutes

Cooking time: 30 minutes

Servings: 1

Ingredients:

- 1/2 cup low fat milk
- 1 egg, beaten
- 1/8 teaspoon nutmeg
- 1/8 teaspoon vanilla
- Sweetener, to taste
- 1/2 cup water

Directions:

1. Slightly warm up the milk in a pan, then whisk in the egg, nutmeg, vanilla and sweetener.
2. Pour this custard mixture into a ramekin.
3. Set the ramekin in a baking pan and pour 1/2 cup water into the pan.
4. Bake the custard for 30 minutes at 325 degrees F.
5. Serve fresh.

Nutrition Facts Per Serving:

Calories: 127 kcal
Total Fat: 7 g
Saturated Fat: 2.9 g
Cholesterol: 174 mg
Carbohydrates: 6.6 g
Sugars: 6 g
Protein: 9.6 g
Phosphorus: 309 mg
Potassium: 171 mg

156. Strawberry Pie

Preparation time: 5 minutes

Cooking time: 25 minutes

Servings: 6

Ingredients:

- 1 unbaked (9 inches) pie shell
- 4 cups strawberries, fresh
- 1 cup of brown Swerve
- 3 tablespoons arrowroot powder
- 2 tablespoons lemon juice
- 4-6 tablespoons whipped cream topping

Directions:

1. Spread the pie shell in the pie pan and bake it until golden brown.
2. Now mash 2 cups of strawberries with the lemon juice, arrowroot powder, and Swerve in a bowl.
3. Add the mixture to a saucepan and cook on moderate heat until it thickens.
4. Allow the mixture to cool then spread it in the pie shell.
5. Slice the remaining strawberries and spread them over the pie filling.
6. Refrigerate for 1 hour then garnish with whipped cream.
7. Serve fresh and enjoy.

Nutrition Facts Per Serving:

Calories: 236 kcal
Total Fat: 11.1 g
Saturated Fat: 3.3 g
Cholesterol: 3mg
Carbohydrate: 26 g
Sugars: 7.5 g
Protein: 2.2 g
Phosphorous: 47.2 mg
Potassium: 178 mg

157. Apple Crisp

Preparation time: 5 minutes

Cooking time: 45 minutes

Servings: 6

Ingredients:

- 4 cups apples, peeled and chopped
- 1/2 teaspoon stevia
- 3 tablespoons brandy
- 2 teaspoons lemon juice
- 1/2 teaspoon cinnamon
- 1/8 teaspoon nutmeg
- 3/4 cup dry oats
- 1/4 cup brown Swerve
- 2 tablespoons flour
- 2 tablespoons butter

Directions:

1. Toss the oats with the flour, butter and brown Swerve in a bowl and keep it aside.

2. Whisk the remaining crisp ingredients in an 8-inch baking pan.
3. Spread the oats mixture over the crispy filling.
4. Bake it for 45 minutes at 350 degrees F in a preheated oven.
5. Slice and serve.

Nutrition Facts Per Serving:

Calories: 214 kcal
Total Fat: 4.8 g
Saturated Fat: 0.8g
Cholesterol: 0 mg
Carbohydrate: 26.2 g
Sugars: 15.7g
Protein: 2.1g
Phosphorous: 348 mg
Potassium: 212 mg

158. Almond Cookies

Preparation time: 5 minutes

Cooking time: 12 minutes

Servings: 24

Ingredients:

- 0.5 cup butter, softened
- 1 cup stevia
- 1 egg
- 3 cups flour
- 1 teaspoon baking soda
- 1 teaspoon almond extract

Directions:

1. Beat the butter with the Swerve in a mixer then gradually stir in the remaining ingredients.
2. Merge well until it forms cookie dough then divide the dough into small balls.
3. Spread each ball into 3/4 inch rounds and place them in a cookie sheet.
4. Poke 2-3 holes in each cookie then bake for 12 minutes at 400 degrees F.

5. Serve.

Nutrition Facts Per Serving:

Calories: 1112.59 kcal
Total Fat: 48.27 g
Carbs: 240.03 g
Protein: 22.57 g
Sodium: 42.55 mg
Cholesterol: 7 mg
Sugars: 3.1g
Phosphorous: 360 mg
Potassium: 390 mg

159. Lime Pie

Preparation time: 10 minutes

Cooking time: 5 minutes

Servings: 8

Ingredients:

- 5 tablespoons butter, unsalted
- 1 1/4 cups breadcrumbs
- 1/4 cup stevia
- 1/3 cup lime juice
- 14 oz. condensed milk
- 1 cup lite or 40% fats heavy whipping cream
- 1 (9 inches) pie shell

Directions:

1. Switch on your gas oven and preheat it to 350 degrees F.
2. Whisk the cracker crumbs with the Swerve and melted butter in a suitable bowl.
3. Spread this cracker crumbs crust in a 9 inches pie shell and bake it for 5 minutes.
4. Meanwhile, mix the condensed milk with the lime juice in a bowl.
5. Whisk the heavy cream in a mixer until foamy, and then add in the condensed milk mixture.
6. Mix well, and then spread this filling in the baked crust.
7. Refrigerate the pie for 4 hours.
8. Slice and serve.

Nutrition Facts Per Serving:

Calories: 391 kcal
Total Fat: 22.4 g

Saturated Fat: 11.5 g

Cholesterol: 57 mg

Total Carbohydrate: 32.9 g

Sugars: 27.4 g

Protein: 5.3 g

Phosphorous: 199 mg

Potassium: 221 mg

160. Buttery Lemon Squares

Preparation time: 5 minutes

Cooking time: 35 minutes

Servings: 12

Ingredients:

- 1 cup refined Swerve
- 1 cup flour
- 1/2 cup butter, unsalted
- 1 cup stevia
- 1/2 teaspoon baking powder
- 2 eggs, beaten
- 4 tablespoons lemon juice
- 1 tablespoon butter, unsalted, softened
- 1 tablespoon lemon zest

Directions:

1. Start mixing 1/4 cup refined Swerve, 1/2 cup butter, and flour in a bowl.
2. Spread this crust mixture in an 8-inch square pan and press it.
3. Bake this flour crust for 15 minutes at 350 degrees F.
4. Meanwhile, prepare the filling by beating 2 tablespoons lemon juice, granulated Swerve, eggs, lemon rind, and baking powder in a mixer.
5. Spread this filling in the baked crust and bake again for about 20 minutes.
6. Meanwhile, prepare the squares' icing by beating 2 tablespoons lemon juice, 1 tablespoon butter, and 3/4 cup refine Swerve.
7. Once the lemon pie is baked well, allow it to cool.

8. Sprinkle the icing mixture on top of the lemon pie then cut it into 36 squares.
9. Serve.

Nutrition Facts Per Serving:

Calories: 229 kcal
Total Fat: 9.5 g
Saturated Fat: 5.8 g
Cholesterol: 50 mg
Carbohydrate: 22.8 g
Sugars: 16 g
Protein: 2.1 g
Phosphorous: 257 mg
Potassium: 51 mg

161. Chocolate Gelatin Mousse

Preparation time: 3 minutes
Preparation time: 5 minutes
Cooking time: 5 minutes
Servings: 4

Ingredients:

- 1 teaspoon stevia
- 1/2 teaspoon gelatin
- 1/4 cup milk
- 1/2 cup dark, unsweetened chocolate chips
- 1 teaspoon vanilla
- 1/2 cup heavy cream, whipped

Directions:

1. Whisk the stevia with the gelatin and milk in a saucepan and cook up to a boil.
2. Stir in the chocolate and vanilla then mix well until it has completely melted.
3. Beat the cream in a mixer until fluffy then fold in the chocolate mixture.
4. Mix it gently with a spatula then transfer to the serving bowl.
5. Refrigerate the dessert for 4 hours.
6. Serve.

Nutrition Facts Per Serving:

Calories: 400 kcal
Total Fat: 12.1 g
Cholesterol: 27 mg
Carbohydrates: 4.7 g

Sugars: 0.8 g

Protein: 3.2 g

Phosphorous: 120 mg

Potassium: 100 mg

162. Blackberry Cream Cheese Pie

Preparation time: 10 minutes

Cooking time: 45 minutes

Servings: 8

Ingredients:

- 1/3 cup butter, unsalted
- 4 cups blackberries
- 1 teaspoon stevia
- 1 cup flour
- 1/2 teaspoon baking powder
- 3/4 cup cream cheese

Directions:

1. Switch your gas oven to 375 degrees F to preheat.
2. Layer a 2-quart baking dish with melted butter.
3. Mix the blackberries with stevia in a small bowl.
4. Beat the remaining ingredients in a mixer until they form a smooth batter.
5. Evenly spread this pie batter in the prepared baking dish and top it with blackberries.
6. Bake the blackberry pie for about 45 minutes in the preheated oven.
7. Slice and serve once chilled.

Nutrition Facts Per Serving:

Calories: 450 kcal

Total Fat: 8.4 g

Saturated Fat: 4.9 g

Cholesterol: 20 mg

Carbohydrate: 26.2 g

Sugars: 15.1 g

Protein: 2.8 g

Phosphorous: 105 mg

Potassium: 170 mg

163. Apple Cinnamon Pie

Preparation time: 5 minutes

Cooking time: 50 minutes

Servings: 12

Ingredients:

Apple Filling:

- 9 cups apples, peeled, cored and sliced
- 1 tablespoon stevia
- 1/3 cup all-purpose flour
- 2 tablespoons lemon juice
- 1 teaspoon ground cinnamon

Pie Dough:

- 2 1/4 cups all-purpose flour
- 1 teaspoon stevia
- 3 tablespoons cold heavy whipping cream
- Water, if needed

Directions:

1. Start by preheating your gas oven at 425 degrees F.
2. Mix the apple slices with cinnamon, lemon juice, flour and stevia in a bowl and keep it aside covered.
3. Whisk the flour with stevia, and cream in a mixing bowl to form the dough.
4. If the dough is too dry, slowly attach some water to make a smooth dough ball.
5. Cut the dough into two equal-size pieces and spread them into a 9-inch sheet.
6. Set one of the sheets at the bottom of a 9-inch pie pan.
7. Evenly spread the apples in this pie shell and add a tablespoon of butter over it.
8. Cover the apple filling with the second sheet of the dough and pinch down the edges.
9. Make 1-inch deep cuts on top of the pie and bake for about 50 minutes until golden.
10. Slice and serve.

Calories: 810.08 kcal

Total Fat: 10.07 g

Cholesterol: 26 mg

Carbs: 170.26 gg

Protein: 18.21 g

Sugars: 31.02 g

Sodium: 9.54 mg

Phosphorous: 220 mg

Potassium: 450 mg

164. Maple Crisp Bars

Preparation time: 5 minutes

Cooking time: 5 minutes

Servings: 20

Ingredients:

- 1/3 cup butter
- 1 cup brown Swerve
- 1 teaspoon maple extract
- 1/2 cup maple syrup
- 8 cups puffed rice cereal

Directions:

1. Mix the butter with Swerve, maple extract, and syrup in a saucepan over moderate heat.
2. Cook by slowly stirring this mixture for 5 minutes then toss in the rice cereal.
3. Mix well, then press this cereal mixture in a 13x9 inches baking dish.
4. Refrigerate the mixture for 2 hours then cut into 20 bars.
5. Serve.

Nutrition Facts Per Serving:

Calories: 180 kcal

Total Fat: 3.1 g

Sodium: 36 mg

Carbohydrate: 10.6g

Sugars: 5.4 g

Protein: 0.4 g

Phosphorus: 233 mg

Potassium: 24 mg

165. Pineapple Gelatin Pie

Preparation time: 5 minutes

Cooking time: 5 minutes

Servings: 8

Ingredients:

- 2/3 cup graham cracker crumbs
- 2 1/2 tablespoons butter, melted
- 1 (20-oz) can crushed pineapple, juice packed
- 1 small gelatin pack
- 1 tablespoon lemon juice
- 2 egg whites, pasteurized
- 1/4 teaspoon cream of tartar

Directions:

1. Whisk the crumbs with the butter in a bowl then spread them onto an 8-inch pie plate.
2. Bake the crust at 425 degrees F.
3. Meanwhile, mix the pineapple juice with the gelatin in a saucepan.
4. Place it over low heat then add the pineapple and lemon juice. Mix well.
5. Whip the cream of tartar and egg whites in a mixer until creamy.
6. Add the cooked pineapple mixture then mix well.
7. Spread this filling in the baked crust.
8. Refrigerate the pie for 4 hours then slice.
9. Serve.

Nutrition Facts Per Serving:

Calories: 180 kcal

Total Fat: 4.2 g

Cholesterol: 0 mg

Carbohydrate: 14.5 g

Sugars: 9.4 g

Protein: 2.2 g

Phosphorous: 10 mg

Potassium: 160 mg

166. Cherry Pie Dessert

> **Preparation time: 5 minutes**
>
> **Cooking time: 40 minutes**
>
> **Servings: 8**

Ingredients:

- 1/2 cup butter, unsalted
- 2 eggs
- 1 cup stevia
- 1 cup sour cream
- 1 teaspoon vanilla
- 2 cups all-purpose flour
- 1 teaspoon baking powder
- 1 teaspoon baking soda
- 20 oz. cherry pie filling

Directions:

1. First, begin by setting your gas oven at 350 degrees F.
2. Soften the butter first, then beat it with the cream eggs, Swerve, vanilla, and sour cream in a mixer.
3. Separately merge the flour with the baking soda and baking powder.
4. Add this mixture to the egg mixture and mix well until smooth.
5. Spread the batter evenly in a 9x13 inch baking pan.
6. Bake the pie for 40 minutes in the oven until golden from the surface.
7. Slice and serve with cherry pie filling on top.

Nutrition Facts Per Serving:

Calories: 470 kcal
Total Fat: 19 g
Cholesterol: 84 mg
Carbohydrate: 43.2 g
Sugars: 14.9 g
Protein: 5.9 g
Phosphorus: 249 mg
Potassium: 232 mg

167. Strawberry Pizza (Healthy, Low Caloric)

Preparation time: 5 minutes

Cooking time: 15 minutes

Servings: 12

Ingredients:

Crust:

- 1 cup flour
- 1/4 cup Swerve
- 1/2 cup butter

Filling:

- 8 oz. cream cheese, softened
- 1/2 teaspoon vanilla
- 3/4 tablespoon stevia
- 2 cups sliced strawberries

Directions:

1. Mix the flour with the Swerve, butter, and enough water to make dough.
2. Spread this dough evenly in a pie pan.
3. Bake the crust at 350 degrees F.
4. Whip the cream cheese with the stevia and vanilla in a mixer until fluffy.
5. Spread this cream cheese filling in the crust and top it with strawberries.
6. Serve.

Nutrition Facts Per Serving:

Calories: 500 kcal

Total Fat: 56.31 g

Carbs: 62.54 g

Sugars: 0.9 g

Protein: 9.95 g

Sodium: 243.31 mg

Dietary Fiber: 1g

Calcium: 25mg

Phosphorous: 154 mg

Potassium: 311 mg

168. Pumpkin Cinnamon Roll

Preparation time: 5 minutes

Cooking time: 15 minutes

Servings: 24

Ingredients:

Dough:

- ½ cups low fat 1% milk
- 1 cup water
- 3 Tbsp olive oil
- ½ cup Swerve brown swerve
- 2 ¼ teaspoons active dry yeast
- ½ cup pumpkin puree
- 2 ½ cups flour
- ¼ teaspoon ground nutmeg
- ½ teaspoon baking soda
- 2 Tbsp butter, melted
- Vegetable oil spray for pans

Filling:
- 1/2 cup butter, melted
- 1/2 cup brown Swerve
- 1/2 cup brown granulated Swerve
- 1/2 teaspoon cinnamon
- 1/2 teaspoon ground ginger
- 1/4 teaspoon ground nutmeg

Directions:

1. Switch on your gas oven and let it preheat at 375 degrees F.
2. Whisk all the ingredients for the dough in a mixing bowl.
3. Spread the dough in a loaf pan into a 1/2-inch layer and bake it for 15 minutes.
4. Meanwhile, whip all the ingredients for the filling in a bowl.
5. Place the baked cake in a serving plate and top it with the prepared filling.
6. Roll the cake and slice it.
7. Serve.

Nutrition Facts Per Serving:

Calories: 915.09 kcal
Total Fat: 34.92 g
Carbs: 129.59 g
Sugars: 5.64 g
Protein: 20.01 g
Sodium: 37.68 mg
Potassium: 370 mg
Phosphorus: 300 mg

169. Peppermint Cookies

Preparation time: 5 minutes

Cooking time: 12 minutes

Servings: 12

Ingredients:

- 2 1/2 cups all-purpose flour
- 1 teaspoon baking soda
- 3/4 cup cocoa powder
- 1 cup butter, unsalted
- 1 cup granulated Swerve
- 1 cup brown Swerve
- 2 large eggs
- 1 teaspoon vanilla extract
- 1/2 teaspoon peppermint extract
- 1 cup of dark, unsweetened chocolate chips
- 1 cup peppermint crunch pieces
- 1/2 cup crushed candies

Directions:

1. Begin by softening the butter at room temperature.
2. Add 12 peppermint candies to a Zip lock bag and crush them using a mallet.
3. Beat the butter with the egg, Swerve, and peppermint extract in a mixer until fluffy.
4. Stir in the baking powder and flour and mix well until smooth.
5. Stir in the crushed peppermint candies and refrigerate the dough for 1 hour.
6. Meanwhile, you can layer a baking sheet with parchment paper.
7. Switch the oven to 350 degrees F to preheat.
8. Now crush the remaining candies and keep them aside.
9. Make 3/4 inch balls out of the dough and place them in the baking sheet.

10. Drizzle the crushed candies over the balls.
11. Bake them for 12 minutes until lightly browned.
12. Serve fresh and enjoy.

Nutrition Facts Per Serving:

Calories: 362 kcal
Total Fat: 16.5 g
Saturated Fat: 10.1 g
Cholesterol: 71 mg
Sodium: 224 mg
Carbohydrates: 31.7 g
Dietary Fiber: 2.5 g
Sugars: 16.9 g
Protein: 5.8 g
Calcium: 25 mg
Phosphorus: 233 mg
Potassium: 138 mg

170. Pumpkin Cheese Pie

Preparation time: 2 minutes

Cooking time: 6 minutes

Servings: 8

Ingredients:

- 1 1/4 cups graham cracker crumbs
- 1/3 cup unsalted butter, melted

Filling:
- 8 oz. cream cheese, softened
- 1/2 cup pumpkin
- 1 teaspoon stevia
- 2 eggs
- 1 teaspoon vanilla
- 1 teaspoon cinnamon
- 1/2 teaspoon nutmeg

Sauce:
- 1 cup water
- 1 tablespoon cornstarch
- 2 teaspoons lemon juice
- 2 cups fresh cranberries

Directions:

1. Blend the cracker crumbs with the butter in a bowl then spread them onto a 9-inch pie plate.
2. Beat the cream cheese with the pumpkin, stevia, egg, cinnamon, nutmeg, vanilla in a mixer.
3. Whisk the water with the lemon juice and cranberries in a saucepan, then cook, stirring slowly until it thickens.
4. Spread the cream cheese filling in the crumbs crust then top it with cranberries sauce.
5. Refrigerate the pie for 4 hours.
6. Slice and serve.

Nutrition Facts Per Serving:

Calories: 831.31 kcal
Total Fat: 75.34 g
Cholesterol: 72 mg
Carbs: 27.82 g
Sodium 563.36 mg
Sugars: 9.38 g

Protein: 14.47 g
Phosphorous: 240 mg
Potassium: 350 mg

171. Ribbon Cakes

Preparation time: 5 minutes
Cooking time: 20 minutes
Servings: 21

Ingredients:

- 1 1/2 cups flour
- 1/2 cup of Swerve
- 1/2 teaspoon baking powder
- 1/2 cup butter, softened
- 1 whole eggs
- 1/2 egg white
- 1/4 teaspoon vanilla
- 1/2 cup jelly
- 1 tablespoon brown Swerve

Directions:

1. Prepare and preheat the oven at 375 degrees F.
2. Whisk the flour with the baking powder and Swerve in a bowl.

3. Beat the butter with cornmeal, eggs, egg white, and vanilla in a beater.
4. Stir in the flour and mix well to form dough.
5. Knead this dough on a floured surface and cut it into 2 equal pieces.
6. Spread each piece into a 1/8-inch thick sheet.
7. Spread one dough layer in an 11x15 inch cookie pan and top it with jelly.
8. Slice the second layer into 1/2-inch wide strips.
9. Place these strips over the jelly and arrange them in a Criss cross manner.
10. Drizzle brown Swerve over the dough then bake for 20 minutes approximately.
11. Cut the baked pie into 1x2 inches rectangles.
12. Serve.

Nutrition Facts Per Serving:

Calories: 160 kcal
Total Fat: 4.7 g
Saturated Fat: 2.9 g
Cholesterol: 19 mg
Sodium: 17 mg
Carbohydrate: 13.6 g
Dietary Fiber: 0.3 g
Sugars: 2.7 g
Protein: 1.3 g
Calcium: 10 mg
Phosphorous: 37 mg
Potassium: 21 mg

172. Raspberry Popsicle

Preparation Time: 2 hours
Cooking Time: 15 minutes
Servings: 4

Ingredients:

- 1 1/2 cups raspberries
- 2 cups of water

Direction:

1. Take a pan and fill it up with water
2. Add raspberries
3. Place it over medium heat and bring to water to a boil
4. Set the heat and simmer for 15 minutes

5. Remove heat and pour the mix into Popsicle molds
6. Add a popsicle stick and let it chill for 2 hours
7. Serve and enjoy!

Nutrition Facts Per Serving:

Calories: 48.02 kcal
Total Fat: 0.6 g
Carbs: 11.03 g
Sugars: 4.08 g
Protein: 1.11 g
Sodium: 5.72 mg
Potassium: 141 mg
Phosphorus: 26 mg

173. Baked Cinnamon Over Apple Raisins

Preparation time: 5 minutes

Cooking time: 5 minutes

Servings: 4

Ingredients:

- 1 tsp. grated lemon peel
- 1/4 cup raisins
- 1/2 tsp. ground cinnamon
- 1/2 cup 100% apple juice
- 2 tbsps. brown sugar
- 1/8 tsp. nutmeg
- 4 cored apples
- 1 tbsp. lemon juice

Directions:

1. Layer apples in a baking dish. Fill them with raisins.
2. Meanwhile, in a small bowl, put together apple juice, nutmeg, lemon juice, ground cinnamon, brown sugar, and lemon peel. Mix ingredients until well-combined.
3. Coat apples with the mixture. Cover with plastic wrap. Set aside.
4. For the remaining cinnamon, place inside the microwave and heat for 4 minutes or until the sauce thickens.
5. Drizzle over apples Serve.

Nutrition Facts Per Serving:

Calories: 390 kcal

Protein: 0.82 g

Potassium: 303 mg

Sodium: 5 mg

Carbs: 40 g

Fat: 2.5 g

Phosphorus: 108.8 mg

174. Banana Cookies

Preparation time: 4 minutes

Cooking time: 26 minutes

Servings: 8

Ingredients:

- 2 tbsps. dried and chopped raisins
- 4 pitted dates
- 3 tbsps. dried and chopped cranberries
- 1/4 cup unsweetened almond milk
- 1 tsp. vanilla
- 1 tsp. baking powder
- 1 tbsp. cinnamon
- 2/3 cup coconut flour
- 2 peeled ripe bananas
- 2/3 cup unsweetened applesauce
- 1 1/2 tsps. lemon juice

Directions:

1. Preheat the oven to 350F.
2. In a food processor, combine almond milk, applesauce, dates, and bananas. Blend until you achieve a smooth consistency.
3. Add in coconut flour, baking powder, cinnamon, vanilla, and lemon juice. Blend for 1 minute. Fold in cranberries and raisins.
4. Pour a baking sheet with the cookie dough. Place inside the oven for 20 minutes.
5. Allow to sit for 5 minutes and let it harden. Serve.

Nutrition Facts Per Serving:

Calories: 481.85 kcal

Total Fat: 6.2 g

Carbs: 107.56 g

Sugars: 64.58 g

Sodium: 296.62 mg

Protein: 1.05 g

Potassium: 590 mg
Sodium: 296.62 mg
Phosphorus: 93 mg

175. Easy Fudge

Preparation Time: 15 minutes + chill time

Cooking Time: 5 minutes

Servings: 25

Ingredients:

- 2 tbsp. of coconut butter
- 1 cup pumpkin puree
- 1 teaspoon ground cinnamon
- 1/4 teaspoon ground nutmeg
- 1 tablespoon coconut oil

Direction:

1. Take an 8x8 inch square baking pan and line it with aluminum foil
2. Take a spoon and scoop out the coconut butter into a heated pan and allow the butter to melt
3. Keep stirring well and remove from the heat once fully melted
4. Add spices and pumpkin and keep straining until you have a grain-like texture
5. Add coconut oil and keep stirring to incorporate everything
6. Scoop the mixture into your baking pan and evenly distribute it
7. Place wax paper on top of the mixture and press gently to straighten the top
8. Remove the paper and discard
9. Allow it to chill for 1-2 hours
10. Once chilled, take it out and slice it up into pieces.

Nutrition Facts Per Serving:

Calories: 214.61 kcal
Fat: 16.83 g
Carbohydrates: 15.17 g
Protein: 2.06 g
Protein: 15.02 g

Sodium: 6 mg

Potassium: 10 mg

Phosphorus: 1.5 mg

176. Choco-Chip Cookies with Walnuts and Oatmeal

Preparation Time: 20 minutes

Cooking Time: 32 minutes

Servings: 48

Ingredients:

- 3 Tbsp walnuts, chopped
- ½ cup whole wheat pastry flour
- ½ tsp baking soda
- ½ cup dark chocolate chip
- 1 egg large
- 1 egg white, medium
- 1 Tbsp vanilla extract
- 1 tsp ground cinnamon
- ½ cups rolled oats, not quick cooking
- 1 cup light brown sugar, packed
- 3 tbsps. unsalted butter cold

Directions:

1. Set two racks, leaving at least a 3-inch space in between them. Preheat the oven to 350F and grease baking sheets with cooking spray.
2. In a medium bowl, whisk together baking soda, cinnamon, whole wheat flour, all-purpose flour and oats. In a large bowl, with a mixer beat butter until well combined. Add brown sugar and granulated sugar, mixing continuously until creamy.
3. Mix in vanilla, egg white and egg and beat for a minute. Merge in the dry Ingredients: until well incorporated. Fold in walnuts and Choco chips. Get a tablespoon full of the batter and roll with your moistened hands into a ball.

4. Evenly place balls into prepared baking sheets at least 2-inches apart bake for 16 minutes. Ten minutes into baking time, switch pans from top to bottom and bottom to top. Continue baking for 6 more minutes.

5. Detach from the oven, cool on a wire rack. Allow pans to cool completely before adding the next batch of cookies to be baked. Cookies can be stored for up to 2-weeks in a tightly sealed container or longer in the ref.

Nutrition Facts Per Serving:

Calories: 1086.47 kcal
Total Fat: 45.55 g
Carbs: 153.09 g
Sugars: 105.35 g
Protein: 17.35 g
Sodium: 97 mg
Potassium: 1200 mg
Phosphorus: 900 mg

177. Pineapple Pudding

Preparation time: 5 minutes
Cooking time: 15 minutes
Servings: 12

Ingredients:

- 3 tablespoons all-purpose flour
- 1 tablespoon brown Swerve
- 4 large eggs
- 1 cup milk
- 1 cup water
- 1 teaspoon vanilla extract
- 2 cups pineapple chunks, drained
- 2 drops liquid stevia
- 30 vanilla wafers

Directions:

1. Prepare and preheat the oven at 425 degrees F.
2. Whisk the flour with 1 whole egg, 3 egg yolks, and Swerve in a bowl.
3. Place this bowl over boiling water and stir in

the vanilla essence, stevia, milk and water.

4. Stir and cook until it thickens.

5. Remove the custard from the heat and spread it in a 1 1/2 quart casserole dish.

6. Top the custard with half of the vanilla wafers and half of the pineapple.

7. Repeat the layers in the same manner.

8. Beat the egg whites with the Swerve in an electric mixer until fluffy.

9. Top the custard casserole with egg white fluff.

10. Bake this custard casserole for 5 minutes in the oven.

11. Serve.

Nutrition Facts Per Serving:

Calories: 337.47 kcal
Total Fat: 11.26 g
Carbs: 49.58 g
Sugars: 32.21 g
Protein: 10.18 g
Sodium: 186.38 mg
Phosphorus: 190 mg
Potassium: 320 mg

Side Dishes

178. Braised Sweet Cabbage

Preparation time: 10 minutes

Cooking time: 10 minutes

Servings: 4

Ingredients:

- 1 small cabbage head, shredded
- 2 tablespoons water
- A drizzle of olive oil
- 6 ounces shallots, cooked and chopped
- A pinch of black pepper
- A pinch of sweet paprika
- 1 tablespoon dill

Directions:

1. Warmth up a pan with the oil over medium heat, add the cabbage and the water, stir and sauté for 5 minutes.
2. Attach the rest of the ingredients, toss, cook for 5 minutes more, divide everything between plates and serve as a side dish!

3. Enjoy!

Nutrition Facts Per Serving:

Calories 91 kcal

Fat 1 g

Fiber 15 g

Carbs 20 g

Protein 4 g

Phosphorus: 120 mg

Potassium: 127 mg

Sodium: 75 mg

179. Cauliflower and Leeks

Preparation time: 10 minutes

Cooking time: 20 minutes

Servings: 4

Ingredients:

- 1 and 1/2 cups leeks, chopped
- 1 and 1/2 cups cauliflower florets
- 2 garlic cloves, minced
- 1 and 1/2 cups artichoke hearts
- 2 tablespoons coconut oil, melted

214

- Black pepper to taste

Directions:

1. Warmth up a pan with the oil over medium-high heat, add garlic, leeks, cauliflower florets and artichoke hearts, stir and cook for 20 minutes.
2. Add black pepper, stir, divide between plates and serve.
3. Enjoy!

Nutrition Facts Per Serving:

Calories: 252.53 kcal
Total Fat: 14.41 g
Fiber: 8 g
Carbs: 29.43
Protein: 6.82 g
Phosphorus: 154.59 mg
Potassium: 683.66 mg
Sodium: 410.59 mg

180. Eggplant and Mushroom Sauté

Preparation time: 10 minutes
Cooking time: 30 minutes
Servings: 4

Ingredients:

- 2 pounds oyster mushrooms, chopped
- 6 ounces shallots, peeled, chopped
- 1 yellow onion, chopped
- 2 eggplants, cubed
- 3 celery stalks, chopped
- 1 tablespoon parsley, chopped
- A pinch of sea salt
- Black pepper to taste
- 1 tablespoon savory, dried
- 3 tablespoons coconut oil, melted

Directions:

1. Warmth up a pan with the oil over medium high heat, adds onion, stir and cook for 4 minutes.
2. Add shallots, stir and cook for 4 more minutes.

3. Add eggplant pieces, mushrooms, celery, savory and black pepper to taste, stir and cook for 15 minutes.
4. Add parsley, stir again, cook for a couple more minutes, divide between plates and serve.
5. Enjoy!

Nutrition Facts Per Serving:

Calories: 514.5 kcal
Total Fat: 23.11 g
Carbs: 70.89 g
Protein: 21.69 g
Sugars: 24.91 g
Sodium: 208.3 mg
Phosphorus: 3285.95 mg
Potassium: 217 mg

181. Mint Zucchini

Preparation time: 10 minutes
Cooking time: 7 minutes
Servings: 4

Ingredients:

- 2 tablespoons mint
- 2 zucchinis, halved lengthwise and then slice into half moons
- 1 tablespoon coconut oil, melted
- 1/2 tablespoon dill, chopped
- A pinch of cayenne pepper

Directions:

1. Warmth up a pan with the oil over medium-high heat, adds zucchinis, stir and cook for 6 minutes.
2. Add cayenne, dill and mint, stir, cook for 1 minute more, divide between plates and serve.
3. Enjoy!

Nutrition Facts Per Serving:

Calories: 120 kcal
Fat 3 g
Fiber 1 g
Carbs 3 g
Protein 1 g
Phosphorus: 120 mg
Potassium: 127 mg
Sodium: 75 mg

182. Celery and Kale Mix

Preparation time: 10 minutes

Cooking time: 20 minutes

Servings: 4

Ingredients:

- 2 celery stalks, chopped
- 3 cups kale, torn
- 1 small red bell pepper, chopped
- 3 tablespoons water
- 1 tablespoon coconut oil, melted

Directions:

1. Warmth up a pan with the oil over medium-high heat, adds celery, stir and cook for 10 minutes.
2. Add kale, water, and bell pepper, stir and cook for 10 minutes more.
3. Divide between plates and serve.
4. Enjoy!

Nutrition Facts Per Serving:

Calories: 128.37 kcal
Total Fat: 7.9 g
Protein: 5.03 g
Sodium: 71.77 mg
Carbs: 11 g
Phosphorus: 117 mg
Potassium: 700 mg

183. Spicy Mushroom Stir-Fry

Preparation Time: 10 minutes

Cooking Time: 12 minutes

Servings: 4

Ingredients:

- 1 cup low-sodium vegetable broth
- 2 tbsps. cornstarch
- 1 tsp. low-sodium soy sauce
- 1/2 tsp. ground ginger
- 1/8 tsp. cayenne pepper
- 2 tbsps. olive oil
- 2 (8-oz.) packages sliced button mushrooms

- 1 red bell pepper, chopped
- 1 jalapeño pepper, minced

Directions:

1. Take a small bowl, and combine the broth, cornstarch, soy sauce, ginger, and cayenne pepper. Then, set aside.
2. After, take a wok (or a heavy skillet) and warm the olive oil over high heat.
3. Then, add the mushrooms and peppers.
4. Stir frying for 3–5 minutes or until the vegetables are tender-crisp.
5. Stir the broth mixture and add it to the wok, and stir-fry for 3–5 minutes longer or until the vegetables are tender and the sauce has thickened.
6. Serve.

Nutrition Facts Per Serving:

Calories: 300kcal
Fats: 16 g

Carbs: 49 g
Protein: 8 g
Sodium: 95 mg
Phosphorus: 55 mg
Potassium: 1460.35 mg

184. Kale, Mushrooms and Red Chard Mix

Preparation time: 10 minutes

Cooking time: 17 minutes

Servings: 4

Ingredients:

- 1/2 pound brown mushrooms, sliced
- 3 cups kale, roughly chopped
- 1 1/2 tablespoons coconut oil
- 3 cups red chard, chopped
- 2 tablespoons water
- Black pepper to taste

Directions:

1. Warmth up a pan with the oil over medium high heat, adds mushrooms,

stir and cook for 5
minutes.

2. Add red chard, kale and
   water, stir and cook for 10
   minutes.
3. Attach black pepper to
   taste, stir and cook 2
   minutes more.
4. Divide between plates and
   serve.
5. Enjoy!

*Nutrition Facts Per
Serving:*

Calories: 173 kcal
Total Fat: 11.27 g
Fiber: 2 g
Carbs: 13.3 g
Protein: 5.4 g
Phosphorus: 250 mg
Potassium: 900 mg
Sodium: 75 mg

185. Bok Choy and Beets

Preparation time: 10 minutes
Cooking time: 30 minutes
Servings: 4

Ingredients:

- 1 tablespoon coconut oil
- 4 cups bok choy, chopped
- 3 beets, cut into quarters
  and thinly sliced
- 2 tablespoons water
- A pinch of cayenne
  pepper

Directions:

1. Set water in a large
   saucepan, add the beets to
   a boil over medium heat,
   cover, and cook for 20
   minutes and drain.
2. Warmth up a pan with the
   oil over medium high
   heat, add the bok choy
   and the water, stir and
   cook for 10 minutes.
3. Add beets and cayenne
   pepper, stir, cook for 2
   minutes more, divide

between plates and serve as a side dish!

4. Enjoy!

Nutrition Facts Per Serving:

Calories: 71 kcal
Fat: 3.7 g
Fiber: 7 g
Carbs: 9 g
Protein: 2.3 g
Phosphorus: 110 mg
Potassium: 390 mg
Sodium: 75 mg

186. Spicy Sweet Potatoes

Preparation time: 10 minutes

Cooking time: 40 minutes

Servings: 4

Ingredients:

- 2 sweet potatoes, peeled and thinly sliced
- 2 teaspoons nutmeg, ground
- 2 tablespoon coconut oil, melted
- Cayenne pepper to taste

Directions:

1. In a bowl, mix sweet potato slices with nutmeg, cayenne, and oil and toss to coat well.
2. Spread these on a lined baking sheet, place in the oven at 350 degrees F and bake for 25 minutes.
3. Flip the potatoes, bake for 15 minutes more, divide between plates and serve as a side dish.
4. Enjoy!

Nutrition Facts Per Serving:

Calories: 350 kcal
Fat: 7.5 g
Fiber: 46 g
Carbs: 4.4 g
Protein: 4 g
Phosphorus: 12 0mg
Potassium: 750 mg
Sodium: 75 g

187. Broccoli and Almonds Mix

Preparation time: 10 minutes

Cooking time: 11 minutes

Servings: 4

Ingredients:

- 1 tablespoon olive oil
- 1 garlic clove, minced
- 1 pound broccoli florets
- 1/3 cup almonds, chopped
- Black pepper to taste

Directions:

1. Warmth up a pan with the oil over medium-high heat, add the almonds, stir, cook for 5 minutes and transfer to a bowl,
2. Heat up the same pan again over medium-high heat, add broccoli and garlic, stir, cover and cook for 6 minutes more.
3. Add the almonds and black pepper to taste, stir, divide between plates and serve.

4. Enjoy!

Nutrition Facts Per Serving:

Calories: 250 kcal
Fat: 7.8 g
Fiber: 8 g
Carbs: 9.5 g
Protein: 4.9 g
Phosphorus: 110 mg
Potassium: 869.36 mg
Sodium: 75 mg

188. Squash and Cranberries

Preparation time: 10 minutes

Cooking time: 30 minutes

Servings: 2

Ingredients:

- 1 tablespoon coconut oil
- 1 butternut squash, peeled and cubed
- 2 garlic cloves, minced
- 1 small yellow onion, chopped
- 12 ounces coconut milk
- 1 teaspoon curry powder

- 1 teaspoon cinnamon powder
- 1/2 cup cranberries

Directions:

1. Spread squash pieces on a lined baking sheet, place in the oven at 425 degrees F, bake for 15 minutes and leave to one side.
2. Warm up a pan with the oil over medium high heat, add garlic and onion, stir and cook for 5 minutes.
3. Add roasted squash, stir and cook for 3 minutes.
4. Add coconut milk, cranberries, cinnamon and curry powder, stir and cook for 5 minutes more.
5. Divide between plates and serve as a side dish!
6. Enjoy!

Nutrition Facts Per Serving:

Calories: 442.72 kcal
Total Fat: 20.96 g
Fiber: 7.3 g
Carbs: 67.94 g

Sugars: 14 g
Protein: 7.42 g
Phosphorus: 110 mg
Potassium: 1200 mg
Sodium: 33.02 mg

189. Creamy Chard

Preparation time: 10 minutes
Cooking time: 10 minutes
Servings: 2

Ingredients:

- Juice of 1/2 lemon
- 12 ounces coconut milk
- 1 bunch chard
- A pinch of sea salt
- Black pepper to taste

Directions:

1. Warmth up a pan for 2 minutes with a puff of oil spray, add chard, stir and cook for 5 minutes.
2. Add lemon juice, a pinch of salt, black pepper, and coconut milk, stir and cook for 5 minutes more.
3. Divide between plates and serve as a side.

4. Enjoy!

Nutrition Facts Per Serving:

Calories: 453 kcal

Fat: 47.4 g

Fiber: 4 g

Carbs: 67 g

Protein: 4.2 g

Phosphorus: 130 mg

Potassium: 1127 mg

Sodium: 85 mg

190. Dill Carrots

Preparation time: 10 minutes

Cooking time: 30 minutes

Servings: 4

Ingredients:

- 1 tablespoon coconut oil, melted
- 2 tablespoons dill, chopped
- 1 pound baby carrots
- 1 tablespoon coconut sugar
- A pinch of black pepper

Directions:

1. Set carrots in a large saucepan, add water to cover, bring to a boil over medium-high heat, cover and simmer for 30 minutes.
2. Drain the carrots, put them in a bowl, add melted oil, black pepper, dill, and the coconut sugar, stir very well, divide between plates and serve.
3. Enjoy!

Nutrition Facts Per Serving:

Calories: 85 kcal

Fat: 3.6 g

Fiber: 3.5 g

Carbs: 13.4 g

Protein: 1 g

Phosphorus: 140 mg

Potassium: 147 mg

Sodium: 65 mg

191. Eggs Creamy Melt

Preparation time: 6 minutes

Cooking time: 4 minutes

Servings: 2

Ingredients:

- 1 tbsp. olive oil
- Italian seasoning
- 1 cup shredded tofu
- 2 beaten eggs

Directions:

1. In a small bowl, merge beaten eggs and Italian seasoning. Sprinkle tofu on top.
2. Heat the olive oil in a pan. Add the egg mixture. Cook for 4 minutes on both sides. Serve.

Nutrition Facts Per Serving:

Calories: 214 kcal
Protein: 15.57 g
Potassium: 216 mg
Sodium: 107 mg
Fat: 16.9 g

Carbs: 1.4 g
Phosphorous: 73 mg

192. Cauliflower Mash

Preparation Time: 5 minutes

Cooking Time: 10 minutes

Servings: 4

Ingredients:

- 2 cups of "leached" potatoes
- 2 cups of cauliflower florets
- 2 tbsp. of softened butter
- 3/4 cup of tepid low-fat milk
- 1 tsp. of ground black pepper

Directions:

1. Cut potatoes into quarters.
2. Break apart cauliflower.
3. Add veggies to a large pot of boiling water.
4. Cook until veggies are tender, about 10 minutes.

5. Remove from heat, and drain.
6. Add milk, butter, and pepper.
7. With an immersion blender, cream veggies.
8. Serve hot.

Nutrition Facts Per Serving:

Calories: 310 kcal
Protein: 10 g
Carbs: 37 g
Sodium: 384.7 mg
Phosphorus: 13.7 mg
Potassium: 414.2 mg

193. Jalapeno Crisp

Note: Don't cook this recipe if your potassium or phosphorus lab levels are above normal

Preparation Time: 10 minutes

Cooking Time: 1 hour 15 minutes

Servings: 20

Ingredients:

- 1/2 cup sesame seeds
- 1/2 cup sunflower seeds
- 1/2 cup flax seeds
- 1/2 cup hulled hemp seeds
- 3 tablespoons Psyllium husk
- 1 teaspoon salt
- 1 teaspoon baking powder
- 2 cups of water

Direction:

1. Preheat your oven to 350 F
2. Take your blender and add seeds, baking powder, salt, and Psyllium husk
3. Blend well until a sand-like texture appears
4. Stir in water and mix until a batter form
5. Allow the batter to rest for 10 minutes until a dough-like thick mixture forms
6. Whip the dough onto a cookie sheet lined with parchment paper
7. Spread it evenly, making sure that it has a thickness of 1/4 inch thick all around

8. Bake for 75 minutes in your oven
9. Remove and cut into 20 spices
10. Allow them to cool for 30 minutes and enjoy!

Nutrition Facts Per Serving:

Calories: 700 kcal
Fat: 73 g
Carbohydrates: 30 g
Protein: 33.76 g
Sodium: 1107.12 mg
Potassium: 1000 mg
Phosphorus: 1200 mg

194. Celeriac Tortilla

Preparation Time: 10 minutes
Cooking Time: 25 minutes
Servings: 4

Ingredients:

- 2 oz. celery root, peeled
- 1 potato, peeled
- 1 tablespoon almond flour
- 1/2 teaspoon salt
- 1 egg, beaten
- 1 teaspoon olive oil

Directions:

1. Place potato and celery root in the tray and bake for 15 minutes at 355F. The baked vegetables should be tender.
2. Then transfer them in the food processor. Blend until smooth.
3. Add salt, almond flour, and egg. Knead the soft dough.
4. Cut the dough into 4 pieces and make the balls.
5. Using the rolling pin roll up the dough balls in the shape of tortillas
6. Heat up olive oil in the skillet.
7. Add the first celeriac tortilla and roast it for 1.5 minutes from each side.
8. Repeat the steps with remaining tortilla balls.
9. Store the cooked tortillas in the towel before serving.

Calories: 163.81 kcal
Total Fat: 6.16 g
Carbs: 22.04 g
Sugars: 1.54 g
Protein: 6.02 g
Sodium: 652.2 mg
Potassium: 590 mg
Phosphorus: 130 mg

195. Caraway Mushroom Caps (Low Caloric)

Preparation Time: 8 minutes
Cooking Time: 25 minutes
Servings: 4

Ingredients:

- 1 teaspoon caraway seeds
- 3 oz. Portobello mushroom caps
- 2 teaspoons butter, softened
- 1/4 teaspoon salt

Directions:

1. Trim and wash mushrooms caps if needed.
2. Preheat the oven to 360F.
3. Churn together butter with salt, and caraway seeds.
4. Fill the mushroom caps with butter mixture and transfer in the tray.
5. Bake Portobello caps for 10 minutes at 355F.

Nutrition Facts Per Serving:

Calories: 45.75kcal
Total Fat: 4 g
Carbs: 1.95 g
Sugars: 0.85 g
Protein: 1.57 g
Sodium: 293.5 mg
Potassium: 151 mg
Phosphorus: 44 mg

196. Stuffed Sweet Potato

| Preparation Time: 10 minutes |
| Cooking Time: 20 minutes |
| Servings: 4 |

Ingredients:

- 2 sweet potatoes
- 1/4 cup Cheddar cheese, shredded
- 2 teaspoons butter
- 1 tablespoon fresh parsley, chopped
- 1/2 teaspoon salt

Directions:

1. Make the lengthwise cut in every sweet potato and bake them for 10 minutes at 360F.
2. After this, scoop 1/2 part of every sweet potato flesh.
3. Fill the vegetables with salt, parsley, butter, and shredded cheese.
4. Return the sweet potatoes in the oven back and bake them for 10 minutes more at 355F.

Nutrition Facts Per Serving:

Calories: 480.85 kcal

Total Fat: 8.64 g

Carbs: 91.9 g

Sugars: 19.06 g

Protein: 10.45 g

Sodium: 924.89 mg

Potassium: 1500 mg

Phosphorus: 270 mg

197. Baked Olives

| Preparation Time: 5 minutes |
| Cooking Time: 11 minutes |
| Servings: 3 |

Ingredients:

- 1 1/2 cup olives
- 1 tablespoon olive oil
- 1 teaspoon dried oregano
- 1/4 teaspoon dried thyme
- 1/3 teaspoon minced garlic
- 1/2 teaspoon salt

Directions:

1. Line the baking tray with baking paper.
2. Arrange the olives in the tray in one layer.
3. Then sprinkle them with olive oil, dried oregano, dried thyme, minced garlic, and salt.
4. Bake olives for 11 minutes at 420F.

Nutrition Facts Per Serving:

Calories: 182.07 kcal

Total Fat: 17.94 g

Carbs: 7.08 g

Sugars: 0.03 g

Protein: 0.93 g

Sodium: 1025.2 mg

Potassium: 19 mg

Phosphorus: 4 mg

198. Sliced Figs Salad

Preparation Time: 10 minutes
Cooking Time: 25 minutes
Servings: 4

Ingredients:

- 1 tablespoon balsamic vinegar
- 1 teaspoon canola oil
- 2 tablespoons almonds, sliced
- 3 figs, sliced
- 2 cups fresh parsley
- 1 cup fresh arugula
- 2 oz. Feta cheese, crumbled
- 1/2 teaspoon salt
- 1/2 teaspoon honey

Directions:

1. Make the salad dressing: mix up together balsamic vinegar, canola oil, salt, and honey.
2. Then put sliced almonds and figs in the big bowl.
3. Chop the parsley and add in the fig mixture too.

4. After this, tear arugula.
5. Combine together arugula with fig mixture.
6. Add salad dressing and shake the salad well.

Nutrition Facts Per Serving:

Calories: 247.92 kcal
Total Fat: 14.37 g
Carbs: 24.71 g
Protein: 8.89 g
Sodium: 943.32 mg
Potassium: 600 mg
Phosphorus: 190 mg

199. Lemon Cucumbers with Dill

Preparation Time: 5 minutes
Cooking Time: 30 minutes
Servings: 3

Ingredients:

- 3 cucumbers
- 3 tablespoons lemon juice
- 3/4 teaspoon lemon zest
- 3 teaspoons dill, chopped
- 1 tablespoon olive oil
- 3/4 teaspoon chili flakes

Directions:

1. Peel the cucumbers and chop them roughly.
2. Place the cucumbers in the big glass jar.
3. Add lemon zest, lemon juice, and dill, olive oil, and chili flakes.
4. Close the lid and shake well.
5. Marinate the cucumbers for 30 minutes.

Nutrition Facts Per Serving:

Calories: 115.93 kcal
Total Fat: 7.64 g
Carbs: 13.05 g
Sugars: 5.71 g
Protein: 2.14 g
Sodium: 6.81 mg
Potassium: 480 mg
Phosphorus: 75 mg

200. Honey Apple Bites

Preparation Time: 10 minutes

Cooking Time: 15 minutes

Servings: 2

Ingredients:

- 1 tablespoon honey
- 1/2 teaspoon ground cardamom
- 2 apples

Directions:

1. Slice the apples into halves and detach the seeds.
2. Then cut the apples into 4 bites more.
3. Place the apple bites in the tray and sprinkle with ground cardamom and honey.
4. Bake apples for 15 minutes at 355F.

Nutrition Facts Per Serving:

Calories: 120.47 kcal
Total Fat: 0.27 g
Carbs: 32.22 g
Sugars: 27 g
Protein: 0.58 g
Sodium: 0.51 mg
Potassium: 172 mg
Phosphorus: 24 mg

201. Cucumber Salad

Preparation Time: 10 minutes

Cooking Time: 15 minutes

Servings: 6

Ingredients:

- 2 cups tomatoes, chopped
- 1 cup cucumbers, chopped
- 1 red onion, chopped
- 1 cup fresh cilantro, chopped
- 1 red bell pepper, chopped
- 2 tablespoons sunflower oil

Directions:

1. In the bowl combine together tomatoes,

cucumbers, onion, fresh cilantro, and bell pepper.

2. Shake the salad mixture well.
3. Then add the sunflower oil.
4. Stir the salad directly before serving.

Nutrition Facts Per Serving:

Calories: 198.08 kcal
Total Fat: 14.62 g
Carbs: 15.74 g
Sugars: 10.04 g
Protein: 3.46 g
Sodium: 18.82 mg
Potassium: 790 mg
Phosphorus: 90 mg

202. Sesame Seeds Escarole

Preparation Time: 10 minutes

Cooking Time: 25 minutes

Servings: 4

Ingredients:

- 1 head escarole
- 1 tablespoon sesame oil
- 1 teaspoon sesame seeds
- 1 teaspoon balsamic vinegar
- 3/4 teaspoon ground black pepper
- 1/4 cup of water

Directions:

1. Chop the escarole roughly.
2. Pour water in the skillet and bring it to boil.
3. Add chopped escarole. Saute it for 2 minutes over the high heat.
4. Then add sesame seeds, sesame oil, balsamic vinegar, and ground black pepper.
5. Mix up well and saute escarole for 1 minute more or until it starts to boil again.

Nutrition Facts Per Serving:

Calories: 118 g
Fat: 8.1 g
Fiber: 8.3 g
Carbs: 9.5 g
Protein: 3.6 g

Sodium: 95 mg

Potassium: 720 mg

Phosphorus: 73 mg

203. Yogurt Eggplants

Preparation Time: 10 minutes

Cooking Time: 18 minutes

Servings: 4

Ingredients:

- 1 cup Plain yogurt
- 1 tablespoon butter
- 1 teaspoon ground black pepper
- 1 teaspoon salt
- 2 eggplants, chopped
- 1 tablespoon fresh dill, chopped

Directions:

1. Heat up butter in the skillet.
2. Toss eggplants in the hot butter. Set them with salt and ground black pepper.
3. Roast the vegetables for 5 minutes over the medium-high heat. Stir them from time to time.
4. After this, add fresh dill and Plain Yogurt. Mix up well.
5. Close the lid and simmer eggplants for 10 minutes more over the medium-high heat.

Nutrition Facts Per Serving:

Calories: 214.14 kcal

Total Fat: 10.19 g

Carbs 27.04 g

Sugars: 18.07 g

Protein: 7.86 g

Sodium: 1227.19 mg

Potassium: 1000 mg

Phosphorus: 200 mg

204. Spiced Tortilla Chips

Preparation Time: 10 minutes

Cooking time: 8 minutes

Servings: 8

Ingredients:

- 4 (12-inch) flour tortillas, cut into wedges
- 4 tablespoons olive oil
- 1/2 teaspoon paprika
- 1/2 teaspoon rosemary seasoning
- 1/2 teaspoon cayenne pepper
- Cheddar cheese

Directions:

1. Begin by switching the oven to 425 degrees F to preheat.
2. Grease the baking sheet with cooking spray.
3. Add all the spices and cheese to a small bowl.
4. Mix well and keep this mixture aside.
5. Cut the tortillas into 8 wedges and coat them with the cheese mixture.
6. Spread them on a baking tray and drizzle the remaining cheese mixture on top.
7. Bake at 350 degrees F.
8. Serve fresh.

Nutrition Facts Per Serving:

Calories: 873.53 kcal

Total Fat: 47.13 g

Carbs: 94.91 g

Protein: 19.68 g

Sodium: 1358.17 mg

Potassium: 32 mg

Phosphorus: 72 mg

205. Tuna Dip

Preparation Time: 10 minutes
Cooking time: 0 minutes
Servings: 20

Ingredients:

- 2 (10 oz.) canned tuna chunks, drained
- 2 (8 oz.) packages cream cheese, softened
- 1 cup Ranch dressing
- 3/4 cup pepper sauce
- 11/2 cups Cheddar cheese
- 1 bunch celery,
- 1 (8 oz.) box chicken-flavored crackers

Directions:

1. Add all the tuna dip ingredients to a salad bowl.
2. Toss them well and refrigerate for 1 hour.
3. Serve.

Nutrition Facts Per Serving:

Calories: 256 kcal
Total Fat: 14.6 g
Saturated Fat: 6.6 g
Cholesterol: 108 mg
Sodium: 461 mg
Carbohydrates: 1.4 g
Sugars: 0.4 g
Protein: 30.2 g
Phosphorus: 147 mg
Potassium: 228 mg

Snacks

206. Cauliflower Patties

> **Preparation Time: 5 minutes**
>
> **Cooking Time: 8 minutes**
>
> **Servings: 4**

Ingredients:

- 2 Eggs
- 2 Egg whites
- 1/2, Onion, diced
- 2 cups Cauliflower, frozen
- 2 tbsp. All-purpose white flour
- 1 tsp. Black pepper
- 1 tbsp. Coconut oil
- 1 tsp. Curry powder
- 1 tbsp. Fresh cilantro

Directions:

1. Moisture vegetables in warm water before cooking.
2. Steam cauliflower over a pan of boiling water for 10 minutes.
3. Blend eggs and onion in a food processor before adding cooked cauliflower, spices, cilantro, flour, and pepper, and blast in the processor for 30 seconds.
4. Heat a skillet on high heat and add oil.
5. Enjoy with a salad.

Nutrition Facts Per Serving:

Calories: 190

Fat: 12 g

Carbs: 15 g

Phosphorus: 193 mg

Potassium: 370 mg

Sodium: 158 mg

Protein: 13 g

207. Turnip Chips

> **Preparation Time: 5 minutes**
>
> **Cooking Time: 50 minutes**
>
> **Servings: 2**

Ingredients:

- 2 Turnips, peeled and sliced
- 1 tbsp. Extra virgin olive oil
- 1 Onion chopped

- 1 clove minced garlic
- 1 tsp. Black pepper
- 1 tsp. Oregano
- 1 tsp. Paprika

Directions:

1. Preheat the oven to 375F. Grease a baking tray with olive oil.
2. Add turnip slices in a thin layer.
3. Dust over herbs and spices with an extra drizzle of olive oil.
4. Bake for 40 minutes. Turning once.

Nutrition Facts Per Serving:

Calories: 136 kcal
Fat: 14 g
Carbs: 30 g
Phosphorus: 50 mg
Potassium: 356 mg
Sodium: 71 mg

208. Mixes of Snack

Preparation Time: 10 minutes
Cooking Time: 1 hours and 15 minutes
Servings: 4

Ingredients:

- 2 tbsp. margarine
- 2 tbsp. Worcestershire sauce
- 3/4 c. garlic powder
- 1/2 tsp. onion powder
- 3 cups Crispix
- 3 cups Cheerios
- 3 cups corn flakes
- 1 cup Kix
- half cup pretzels
- half cup broken bagel chips into 1-inch pieces

Directions:

1. Preheat the oven to 250F
2. Melt the margarine in a large roasting pan. Stir in the seasoning. Gradually add the ingredients remaining by mixing so that the coating is uniform.

238

3. Cook for 1 hour, stirring every 15 minutes. Spread on paper towels to let cool. Store in a tightly closed container.

Nutrition Facts Per Serving:

Calories: 1108.52 kcal
Total Fat: 20.16 g
Carbs: 295 g
Sugars: 26.34 g
Protein: 31.8 g
Sodium: 979.75 mg
Potassium: 900 mg
Phosphorus: 540 mg

209. Healthy Cashew and Almond Butter

Preparation Time: 5 minutes
Cooking Time: 0 minutes
Servings: 2

Ingredients:

- 1 cup almonds, blanched
- 1/3 cup cashew nuts
- 2 tablespoons coconut oil
- Salt as needed
- 1/2 teaspoon cinnamon

Direction:

1. Preheat your oven to 350 F
2. Bake almonds and cashews for 12 minutes
3. Let them cool
4. Set to a food processor and add remaining ingredients
5. Add oil and keep blending until smooth
6. Serve and enjoy!

Nutrition Facts Per Serving:

Calories: 679.68 kcal
Total Fat: 62.16 g
Carbs: 21.52 g
Sugars: 4.51 g
Protein: 19.03 g
Sodium: 405.07 mg
Potassium: 620 mg
Phosphorus: 400 mg

210. Veggie Fritters

Preparation Time: 10 minutes
Cooking Time: 10 minutes
Servings: 8

Ingredients:

- 2 garlic cloves, minced
- 2 yellow onions, chopped
- 4 scallions, chopped
- 2 carrots, grated
- 2 teaspoons cumin, ground
- 1/2 teaspoon of turmeric powder
- Salt and black pepper to the taste
- 1/4 teaspoon of coriander, ground
- 2 tablespoons of parsley, chopped
- 1/4 teaspoon of lemon juice
- 1/2 cup of almond flour
- 2 beets, peeled and grated
- 2 eggs, whisked
- 1/4 cup of tapioca flour
- 3 tablespoons of olive oil

Directions:

1. In a bowl, combine the garlic with the onions, scallions, and the rest of the ingredients except the oil, stir well and shape medium fritters out of this mix.

2. Warm up a pan with the oil over medium-high heat, add the fritters, cook for 5 minutes on each side, arrange on a platter, and serve.

Nutrition Facts Per Serving:

Calories: 571.42 kcal
Total Fat: 38.63 g
Carbs: 46.96 g
Protein: 48 g
Sodium: 568.8 mg
Potassium: 1063 mg
Phosphorus: 217 mg

211. Cucumber Bites

Preparation Time: 10 minutes

Cooking Time: 0 minutes

Servings: 12

Ingredients:

- 1 English cucumber, sliced into 32 rounds
- 10 ounces hummus
- 16 cherry tomatoes, halved
- 1 tablespoon of parsley, chopped
- 1 ounce feta cheese, crumbled

Directions:

1. Spread the hummus on each cucumber round, divide the tomato halves on each, sprinkle the cheese and parsley on to, and serve as an appetizer.

Nutrition Facts Per Serving:

Calories: 313.02 kcal
Total Fat: 17.05 g
Carbs: 29.84 g
Sugars: 5.26 g
Protein: 15.12 g
Sodium: 708.54 mg
Potassium: 800 mg
Phosphorus: 350 mg

212. Artichoke Flatbread

Preparation Time: 10 minutes

Cooking Time: 15 minutes

Servings: 4

Ingredients:

- 5 tablespoons olive oil
- 2 garlic cloves, minced
- 2 tablespoons parsley, chopped
- 2 round whole wheat flatbreads
- 1/2 cup mozzarella cheese, grated
- 14 ounces canned artichokes, drained and quartered
- 1 cup baby spinach, chopped
- 1/2 cup cherry tomatoes, halved

- 1/2 teaspoon basil, dried
- Salt and black pepper to the taste

Directions:

1. In a bowl, mix the parsley with the garlic and 4 tablespoons oil, whisk well, and spread this over the flatbreads.
2. Sprinkle the mozzarella.
3. In a bowl, mix the artichokes with the spinach, tomatoes, basil, salt, pepper, and the rest of the oil, toss and divide over the flatbreads as well.
4. Arrange the flatbreads on a baking sheet and bake for 15 minutes.
5. Serve as an appetizer.

Nutrition Facts Per Serving:

Calories: 689.22 kcal
Total Fat: 48.59 g
Carbs: 47.84 g
Protein: 16.27 g
Sodium: 1256.87 mg
Potassium: 230 mg
Phosphorus: 130 mg

213. Red Pepper Tapenade

Preparation Time: 10 minutes
Cooking Time: 10 minutes
Servings: 4

Ingredients:

- 7 ounces roasted red peppers, chopped
- 1/2 cup cheddar, grated
- 1/3 cup parsley, chopped
- 14 ounces low-sodium artichokes, drained and chopped
- 3 tablespoons olive oil
- 1/4 cup capers, drained
- 1 and 1/2 tablespoons lemon juice
- 2 garlic cloves, minced

Directions:

1. In your blender, combine the red peppers with the cheddar and the rest of the ingredients and pulse well.
2. Divide into cups and serve as a snack.

Calories: 360.24 kcal

Total Fat: 26.64 g

Carbs: 18.17 g

Sugars: 5.33 g

Protein: 9.61 g

Sodium: 1575.77 mg

Potassium: 104 mg

Phosphorus: 150 mg

214. Healthy, Coriander Falafel

Preparation Time: 10 minutes

Cooking Time: 10 minutes

Servings: 8

Ingredients:

- 1 cup canned garbanzo beans
- 1 bunch parsley leaves
- 1 yellow onion, chopped
- 5 garlic cloves, minced
- 1 teaspoon coriander, ground
- A pinch of salt and black pepper
- 1/4 teaspoon cayenne pepper
- 1/4 teaspoon baking soda
- 1/4 teaspoon cumin powder
- 1 teaspoon lemon juice
- 3 tablespoons tapioca flour
- Olive oil for topping

Directions:

1. In your food processor, combine the beans with the parsley, onion, and the rest of the ingredients except the oil and the flour and pulse well.
2. Transfer the mix to a bowl, add the flour, stir well, shape 16 balls out of this mix and flatten them a bit.
3. Top the falafels with olive oil and bake them for 5 minutes on each side, arrange them on a platter and serve as an appetizer.

Nutrition Facts Per Serving:

Calories: 201.08kcal

Fat: 3 g

Carbs: 37.89 g

Protein: 8.63 g

Sodium: 440.81 mg

Potassium: 600 mg

Phosphorus: 190 mg

215. Red Pepper Hummus

Preparation Time: 10 minutes

Cooking Time: 0 minutes

Servings: 6

Ingredients:

- 6 ounces roasted red peppers, peeled and chopped
- 16 ounces canned chickpeas, drained and rinsed
- 1/4 cup Greek yogurt
- 3 tablespoons tahini paste
- Juice of 1 lemon
- 3 garlic cloves, minced
- 1 tablespoon olive oil
- A pinch of salt and black pepper
- 1 tablespoon parsley, chopped

Directions:

1. In your food processor, combine the red peppers with the rest of the ingredients except the oil and the parsley and pulse well.
2. Add the oil, pulse again, divide into cups, sprinkle the parsley on top, and serve as a party spread.

Nutrition Facts Per Serving:

Calories: 500.3 kcal

Total Fat: 27.78 g

Carbs 47.78 g

Protein: 19.17 g

Sodium: 887.93 mg

Potassium: 500 mg

Phosphorus: 480 mg

216. Sweet and Sour Beet Dip

> **Preparation Time: 10 minutes**
> **Cooking Time: 50 minutes**
> **Servings: 6**

Ingredients:

- 1-pound beets, trimmed
- 1/2 cup tahini
- 1/2 cup freshly squeezed lemon juice
- 4 garlic cloves, mashed
- Grated zest of 1 lemon
- 1 teaspoon ground cumin
- 1/4 teaspoon cayenne pepper
- Pinch of Salt
- Freshly ground black pepper

Directions:

1. Mix the beets with enough water and then cover. Place the pan on high heat and boil the beets for about 50 minutes or until tender.
2. Drain the beets, let them cool, and peel them. The skins should slide off easily.
3. Transfer the beets to a food processor and purée for about 5 minutes until smooth. Transfer the puréed beets to a medium bowl.
4. Stir in the tahini, lemon juice, garlic, lemon zest, cumin, and cayenne until well mixed. Taste and then season it with some salt and black pepper, as needed.

Nutrition Facts Per Serving:

Calories 582.66kcal
Total Fat 40.51g
Carbs 47.61g
Sugars 17.07g
Protein 18.6g
Sodium 189.81mg
Potassium 1300mg
Phosphorus 600mg

217. Marinated Olives

Preparation Time: 10 minutes

Cooking Time: 0 minutes

Servings: 4

Ingredients:

- 1/4 cup olive oil
- 1/4 cup white wine vinegar
- Grated zest of 1 lemon
- 1 teaspoon chopped fresh rosemary
- 2 cups jarred olives, drained

Directions:

1. Whisk the olive oil, vinegar, lemon zest, and rosemary until blended.
2. Add the olives and gently stir to coat. Put well and let it marinate for at least 3 hours before serving.

Nutrition Facts Per Serving:

Calories 414.03 kcal
Total Fat 42.88 g
Carbs: 9.05 g
Sodium: 991.06 mg
Potassium: 29 mg
Phosphorus: 10 mg

218. Marinated Zucchini

Preparation Time: 15 minutes

Cooking Time: 5 minutes

Servings: 6

Ingredients:

- 1/4 cup balsamic vinegar
- 2 tablespoons stone-ground mustard
- 1 garlic clove, minced
- 2 teaspoons chopped fresh thyme
- 1/4 cup olive oil
- 1/8 teaspoon salt
- 1/8 teaspoon freshly ground black pepper
- 3 large zucchinis, cut diagonally into 1/2-inch-thick slices

Directions:

1. Whisk the vinegar, mustard, garlic, and thyme

to combine. Whisk in the olive oil until blended. Flavor with the salt and pepper and whisk again to combine.

2. Place the zucchini in a large bowl and drizzle 1/4 cup of marinade over them. Toss well to coat.

3. Warmth a grill pan or sauté pan over medium heat.

4. Transfer the cooked zucchini back to the bowl and drizzle it with the remaining marinade. Toss to coat. Cover the bowl and refrigerate the zucchini to marinate for 30 minutes or until chilled.

5. Arrange the marinated slices on a serving platter and drizzle with the marinade from the bowl to serve.

Nutrition Facts Per Serving:

Calories: 366.47 kcal
Total Fat: 29.47 g

Carbs: 21.98 g
Sugars: 15.43 g
Protein: 3.87 g
Sodium: 441.13 mg
Potassium: 800 mg
Phosphorus: 121 mg

219. Pickled Turnips

Preparation Time: 15 minutes

Cooking Time: 0 minutes

Servings: 12

Ingredients:

- 4 cups of water
- 1/4 cup of salt
- 1 cup of white distilled vinegar
- 1 small beet, peeled and quartered
- 1 garlic clove, peeled
- 2 pounds turnips, peeled, halved, and cut into 1/4-inch half-moons

Directions:

1. In a medium bowl, whisk the water and salt until the salt dissolves. Whisk in the vinegar.

247

2. Place the beet and garlic in a clean 2-quart glass jar with a tight-sealing lid. Layer the turnips on top.
3. Pour the vinegar mixture over the turnips to cover them. Seal the lid tightly and let the jar sit at room temperature for 1 week.

Nutrition Facts Per Serving:

Calories: 157.57 kcal
Total Fat: 0.53 g
Carbs: 33.61 g
Sugars: 20.05 g
Protein: 4.84 g
Sodium: 1490.21 mg
Potassium: 1000 mg
Phosphorus: 134 mg

220. Kale Chips

Preparation time: 20 minutes

Cooking time: 25 minutes

Servings: 6

Ingredients:

- 2 cups Kale
- 2 tablespoon olive oil
- 1/4 tablespoon chili powder
- Pinch cayenne pepper

Directions:

1. Preheat the oven to 300F.
2. Set 2 baking sheets with parchment paper; put aside.
3. Remove the stems from the kale and tear the leaves into 2-inch pieces.
4. Wash the kale and dry it thoroughly.
5. Transfer the kale to an outsized bowl and drizzle with vegetable oil.
6. With your hands to toss the kale with oil, taking care to coat each leaf evenly.
7. Season the kale with flavorer and cayenne pepper and toss to mix thoroughly.
8. Spread the seasoned kale in a single layer on each baking sheet. Don't overlap the leaves.
9. Bake the kale, rotating the pans once, for 20 to 25

248

minutes until it's crisp and dry.

10. Remove the trays from the oven and permit the chips to chill on the trays for five minutes.

11. Serve.

221. Tortilla Chips

Preparation time: 15 minutes

Cooking time: 10 minutes

Servings: 6

Ingredients:

- 2 tablespoon brown granulated sugar
- 1/2 tablespoon ground cinnamon
- Pinch ground nutmeg
- 3 (6-inch) whole wheat tortillas
- Cooking spray

Directions:

1. Preheat the oven to 350F.
2. Line a baking sheet with parchment paper.
3. In a small bowl, merge together the sugar, cinnamon, and nutmeg.
4. Set the tortillas on a clean surface and spray each side of every lightly with cooking spray.
5. Sprinkle the cinnamon sugar evenly over each side of every tortilla.
6. Cut the tortillas into 16 wedges each and place them on the baking sheet.
7. Bake the tortilla wedges, turning once, for about 10 minutes or until crisp.
8. Cool the chips

Carb: 9 g

Phosphorus: 29 mg

Potassium: 24 mg

Sodium: 103 mg

Protein: 1 g

222. Buffalo Cauliflower Bites with Dairy-free Ranch Dressing

Preparation time: 15 minutes

Cooking time: 30 minutes

Servings: 8

Ingredients:

- 4 cups cauliflower florets
- 2 tablespoons extra virgin olive oil
- 1/4 teaspoon salt
- 1/4 teaspoon smoked paprika
- 1/4 teaspoon garlic powder
- 1/2 cup sugar-free hot sauce, I used Archie Moore's brand
- 1 tsp. Dairy-free ranch dressing
- 1 tsp. 40% organic mayonnaise
- 0.25 cup silk unsweetened coconut milk
- 1 teaspoon garlic powder
- 1 teaspoon onion powder
- 1/4 teaspoon pepper
- 1 tablespoon fresh lemon juice
- 1/4 cup fresh chopped parsley

Directions:

1. First heat oven to 400F. Spray baking sheet with nonstick vegetable-oil cooking spray. Place florets in a large bowl and toss with vegetable oil. In a small bowl, merge the salt, paprika, and garlic powder with sauce. Add the recent sauce into the cauliflower bowl and stir well until well coated. Scatter cauliflower out evenly on a baking sheet and bake for a half-hour. Whisk

250

the remainder of the ingredients and pour it into a Mason jar. Cover and refrigerate until able to serve with cauliflower bites.

Nutrition Facts Per Serving:

Calories: 289.96 kcal
Total Fat: 23.41 g
Carbs: 17.78 g
Sugars: 7.45 g
Protein: 6.36 g
Sodium: 1892.38 mg
Potassium: 620 mg
Phosphorus: 116 mg

223. Baked Cream Cheese Crab Dip

Preparation time: 5 minutes

Cooking time: 30 minutes

Servings: 12

Ingredients:

- 8 ounces lump crab meat
- 8 ounces cream cheese softened
- 1/2 cup avocado mayonnaise
- 1 tablespoon lemon juice
- 1 teaspoon Worcestershire sauce
- 1/2 teaspoon garlic powder
- 1/2 teaspoon onion powder
- 1/4 teaspoon dry mustard
- 1/4 teaspoon black pepper

Directions:

1. Add all ingredients into a small baking dish and open up evenly. Bake at 375°F for about 25 to half-hour. Serve with low carb crackers or vegetables. Enjoy.

Nutrition Facts Per Serving:

Calories: 683.52 kcal
Total Fat: 57.89 g
Carbs: 10.64 g
Protein: 28.05 g
Sodium: 1939.62 mg
Potassium: 201 mg
Phosphorus: 131 mg

224. Philly Cheese Steak Stuffed Mushrooms

Preparation Time: 15 minutes

Cooking Time: 15 minutes

Servings: 2

Ingredients:

- 24 ounces baby Bella mushrooms
- 1 cup chopped red pepper
- 1 cup chopped onion
- 0.5 tablespoon butter
- ½ teaspoon salt divided
- 1/2 teaspoon pepper divided
- Half pound beef sirloin shaved or thinly sliced against the grain
- 4 ounces provolone cheese

Directions:

1. First heat oven to 350F. Detach stems from mushrooms and place mushrooms on a greased baby sheet. Sprinkle 1/2 teaspoon of salt and 1/4 teaspoon of pepper on each side and bake for a quarter-hour. Set aside. Dissolve 1 tablespoon butter in a large skillet and cook pepper and onions until soft. Then season with 1/2 teaspoon of salt and 1/4 teaspoon of pepper.

2. Remove from the skillet and put aside. In the same skillet, dissolve the remaining tablespoon of butter and attach the meat.

3. Attach the provolone cheese and stir until completely melted.

4. Return the veggies. Add mixture into the mushrooms, top with more cheese if you wish, and bake for five minutes. Serve and luxuriate in.

Nutrition Facts Per Serving:

Calories 649.36kcal

Total Fat 42.06g

Carbs 23.9g

Sugars 13.25g

Protein 49.74g

Sodium 900.89mg

potassium 1600mg

phosphorus 800mg

225. Greek Cookies

Preparation time: 20 minutes

Cooking time: 25 minutes

Servings: 6

Ingredients:

- 1/2 cup Plain yogurt
- 1/2 teaspoon baking powder
- 2 tablespoons Erythritol
- 1 teaspoon almond extract
- 1/2 teaspoon ground clove
- 1/2 teaspoon orange zest, grated
- 3 tablespoons walnuts, chopped
- 1 cup wheat flour
- 1 teaspoon butter, softened
- 1 tablespoon honey
- 3 tablespoons water

Directions:

1. In the bowl, mix the plain yogurt, leaven, Erythritol, flavorer, ground cloves, orange peel, flour, and butter.
2. Knead the non-sticky dough. Add vegetable oil if the dough is too sticky and knead it well.
3. Then make the log from the dough and cut it into small pieces.
4. Roll each piece of dough into the balls and transfer it in the lined with baking paper tray.
5. Press the balls gently and bake for 25 minutes at 350°F.
6. Meanwhile, heat up together honey and water. Simmer the liquid for 1 minute and take away from the warmth.
7. When the cookies are cooked, remove them from the oven and cool for five minutes.

8. Then pour the cookies with sweet honey water and sprinkle with walnuts.
9. Cool the cookies.

Total Fat: 12.46 g
Carbs: 74.42 g
Sodium: 154.33 mg

Nutrition Facts Per Serving:

Calories: 399.29 kcal

Potassium: 240 mg
Phosphorus: 192 mg
Protein: 4.3 g

Salad

226. Salad with Strawberries and Feta Cheese

Preparation time: 20 minutes
Cooking time: 0 minute
Servings: 2

Ingredients:

- Baby lettuce, to taste
- 1-pint strawberries
- Balsamic vinegar
- 2 tbsp Extra virgin olive oil
- 1/4 teaspoon black pepper
- 2-ounces feta cheese

Directions:

1. Prepare the lettuce by washing and drying it, and then cut the strawberries.
2. Cut the feta cheese into 8 pieces.
3. Put together the balsamic vinegar and the extra virgin olive oil in a large cup with a whisk.
4. Mix the strawberries pressing them and putting them in a bowl, add the dressing and mix, then divide the lettuce into four dishes and cut the other strawberries, arranging them on the salad.
5. Put cheese slices on top and add pepper. Serve and enjoy!

Nutrition Facts Per Serving:

Calories: 300 kcal

Fat: 27 g

Protein: 13 g

Sodium: 285 mg

Potassium: 400 mg

Phosphorus: 106 mg

227. Salad with Lemon Dressing

Preparation Time: 10 minutes

Cooking Time: 0 minutes

Servings: 4

Ingredients:

- Heavy cream 1/4 cup
- Freshly squeezed lemon juice 1/4 cup
- Brown sugar 2 Tbsps.
- Chopped fresh dill 2 Tbsps.
- Finely chopped scallion 2 Tbsps. Green part only
- Ground black pepper 1/4 tsp.
- English cucumber 1, sliced thin
- Shredded green cabbage 2 cups

Directions:

1. Get a small bowl, inside which combine the lemon juice, cream, sugar, dill, scallion, and pepper, and mix them well.

2. Next, take a large bowl and combine the cucumber and cabbage.

3. Place the salad in the refrigerator and chill for 1 hour.

4. Mix well before serving.

Nutrition Facts per Serving:

Calories: 110 kcal

Fat: 6 g

Carbs: 13 g

Phosphorus: 38 mg

Potassium: 200 mg

Sodium: 14 mg

Protein: 2 g

228. Barley Blueberry Salad

Preparation Time: 15 minutes

Cooking Time: 25 minutes

Servings: 4

Ingredients:

- 1 cup quick-cooking barley
- 3 cups low-sodium vegetable broth

- 3 tbsps. extra-virgin olive oil
- 2 tbsps. freshly squeezed lemon juice
- 1 tsp. yellow mustard
- 1 tsp. honey
- 1 cup blueberries
- 1/4 cup crumbled feta cheese

Directions:

1. Combine the barley and vegetable broth in a medium saucepan and bring to a simmer.
2. Reduce the heat to low, partially cover the pan, and simmer for 10-12 minutes or until the barley is tender.
3. Meanwhile, whisk together the olive oil, lemon juice, mustard, and honey in a serving bowl until blended.
4. Drain the barley if necessary and add to the bowl. Toss to combine. Wait to be medium-cold.
5. Add the blueberries and feta and toss gently. Serve.

Nutrition Facts Per Serving:

Calories: 345 kcal

Fats: 16 g

Carbs: 44 g

Protein: 7 g

Sodium: 259 mg

Potassium: 301 mg

Phosphorus: 152 mg

229. Salad with Vinaigrette

Preparation Time: 25 minutes

Cooking Time: 0 minutes

Servings: 4

Ingredients:

For the vinaigrette:

- Olive oil 1/2 cup
- Balsamic vinegar 4 Tbsps.
- Chopped fresh oregano 2 Tbsps.
- Pinch red pepper flakes
- Ground black pepper

For the salad:

- Shredded green leaf lettuce 4 cups
- Carrot 1, shredded

- Fresh green beans 3/4 cup, cut into 1-inch pieces
- Large radishes 3, sliced thin

Directions:

1. First, make the vinaigrette by combining its ingredients in a bowl and whisking vigorously.
2. Next, move on to making the salad, mixing the carrot, lettuce, green beans, and radishes in a bowl.
3. At this point, add the vinaigrette to the vegetables and mix well so that the flavors blend.
4. Arrange the salad on plates and serve.

Nutrition Facts Per Serving:

Calories: 586.53 kcal
Fat: 57.9 g
Carbs: 17.12 g
Sugars: 8.56 g
Phosphorus: 58 mg
Potassium: 480 mg
Sodium: 58.81 mg

Protein: 2.84 g

230. Chicken and Mandarin Salad

Preparation Time: 40 minutes
Cooking Time: 30 minutes
Servings: 3

Ingredients:

- 2 Chicken breast halves
- 1/2 cup Celery
- 1/2 cup Green pepper
- 1/4 cup Onion, finely sliced
- 1/4 cup Light mayonnaise
- 1/2 tsp. freshly ground pepper

Directions:

1. Hurl chicken, celery, green pepper, and onion to blend. Include mayo and pepper. Blend delicately and serve.

Nutrition Facts Per Serving:

Calories: 617.37 kcal
Total Fat: 35.31 g

Carbs: 4.23 g

Sugars: 2.03 g

Protein: 65.34 g

Sodium: 461.02 mg

Potassium: 800 mg

Phosphorus: 500 mg

231. Lemony Lentil Salad with Salmon

Preparation Time: 10 minutes

Cooking Time: 0 minutes

Servings: 3

Ingredients:

- 1/4 tsp. salt
- 1/2 cup chopped red onion
- 1 cup diced seedless cucumber
- 1 medium red bell pepper, diced
- 1/3 cup extra virgin olive oil
- 1/3 cup fresh dill, chopped
- 1/3 cup lemon juice
- 2 oz cans of lentils
- 3 oz of salmon, drained and flaked

- 2 tsp. Dijon mustard
- Pepper to taste

Directions:

1. In a bowl, mix lemon juice, mustard, dill, salt, and pepper. Gradually add the oil, bell pepper, onion, cucumber, salmon flakes, and lentils. Toss to coat evenly.

Nutrition Facts Per Serving:

Calories: 496.21 kcal

Total Fat: 44.22 g

Carbs: 14.09 g

Sugars: 6.08 g

Protein: 12.54 g

Sodium: 336.42 mg

Potassium: 517 mg

Phosphorus: 139 mg

232. Pear and Brie Salad

Preparation Time: 15 minutes
Cooking Time: 0 minutes
Servings: 4

Ingredients:

- 1 tbsp. olive oil
- 1 cup arugula
- 1/2 lemon
- 1/2 cup pears
- 1/4 cucumber
- 1/4 cup chopped brie

Directions:

1. Peel and dice the cucumber.
2. Dice the pear.
3. Wash the arugula.
4. Combine salad in a serving bowl and crumble the brie over the top.
5. Whisk the olive oil and lemon juice together.
6. Drizzle over the salad.
7. Season with a little black pepper to taste and serve immediately.

Nutrition Facts Per Serving:

Calories: 100kcal

Protein: 1 g

Carbs: 12 g

Fat: 7 g

Sodium 57 mg

Potassium 115 mg

Phosphorus: 67 mg

233. Cabbage Slaw

Preparation Time: 15 minutes
Cooking Time: 15 minutes
Servings: 2

Ingredients:

- 1 cup shredded green cabbage
- 2/3 cup shredded red cabbage
- 2/3 cup shredded carrots
- 2 tablespoons + 2 teaspoons cilantro (washed and chopped)
- 11/3 tablespoons freshly squeezed lime juice
- 1 tablespoon olive oil

Directions:

1. Merge all ingredients in a bowl and toss together until well mixed.
2. Note: Prepare this slaw about 1–2 hours earlier from the cabbage to soften and flavors to come together.

Nutrition Facts Per Serving:

Calories 145kcal.
Total Fat: 7.2 g
Cholesterol: 0
Sodium: 38.7 mg
Total Carbohydrate: 8.2 g
Dietary Fiber: 2.5 g
Protein: 1.2 g
Iron: 0.5 mg
Potassium: 252.5 mg
Phosphorus: 31 mg

234. Chicken and Pasta Salad

Preparation Time: 30 minutes
Cooking Time: 25 minutes
Servings: 6

Ingredients:

- Chicken Pasta Salad:
- 1 oz. cooked chicken
- 1 cups pasta, spiral, cooked
- 1/2 green pepper, minced
- 1 1/2 tbsp. onion
- 1/2 cup celery
- Garlic Mustard Vinaigrette:
- 2 tbsp. cider Vinegar
- 2 tsp. mustard, prepared
- 1/2 tsp. white sugar
- 1 garlic clove, Minced
- 1/3 cup water
- 1/3 cup olive oil
- 2 tsp. cheddar cheese, grated
- 1/2 tsp. ground pepper

Directions:

1. Combine all the chicken pasta salad ingredients.
2. In a little bowl, combine vinegar, mustard, sugar, garlic, and water slowly in oil. Mix in cheddar. Season with pepper. Join 1/3 measure of dressing with chicken pasta salad and chill.

Nutrition Facts Per Serving:

Calories: 583.64 kcal
Total Fat: 42.88 g
Carbs: 38.8 g
Protein: 11.03 g
Sodium: 160.67 mg
Potassium: 290 mg
Phosphorus: 154 mg

235. Broccoli and Apple Salad

Preparation Time: 15 minutes
Cooking Time: 15 minutes
Servings: 4

Ingredients:

- 3 tablespoons low-fat plain Greek yogurt
- 2 tablespoons lite mayonnaise
- 1 1/2 teaspoons honey
- 1 1/2 teaspoons apple cider vinegar
- 1 cup fresh broccoli florets
- 1/4 medium apple
- 2 tablespoons diced red onion
- 1 tablespoon fresh parsley
- 2 tablespoons dried sweetened cranberries
- 1 tablespoon walnuts

Directions:

1. Trim and cut broccoli florets into small bite-size pieces. Dice the 1/4 apple

into small bite-size pieces. Chop the parsley.

2. Whisk the yogurt, mayonnaise, honey, vinegar, and parsley together in a large bowl.
3. Add the remaining ingredients into the bowl and coat with the yogurt mixture.
4. Refrigerate to chill and let the flavors combine. Stir immediately before serving. (Optional)

Nutrition Facts Per Serving:

Calories: 201.81 kcal
Total Fat: 14.44 g
Carbs: 20.68 g
Sugars: 16.15 g
Protein: 2.99 g
Sodium: 93.79 mg
Potassium: 240 mg
Phosphorus: 74 mg

236. Pasta Salad

Preparation Time: 15 minutes
Cooking Time: 15 minutes
Servings: 4

Ingredients:

- 1/4 tablespoon finely minced onions
- 1/4 cup shredded carrots
- 1/4 cup broccoli florets
- 1/4 cup diced cucumber
- 1/4 cup chopped red bell pepper
- 2 tablespoons distilled white vinegar
- 2 tablespoons olive oil
- A pinch garlic powders
- A pinch black pepper
- 1/8 teaspoon dried oregano
- 1/8 teaspoon celery seed
- 2 ounces rotini pasta
- 1 tablespoon grated Parmesan cheese
- 1/4 teaspoon herb seasoning blend
- A pinch paprika

Directions:

1. Cut broccoli florets into small pieces. Set aside.
2. To make the dressing, combine vinegar, oregano, oil, pepper, garlic powder, celery seed, and onion. Set aside.
3. Cook pasta al dente.
4. Drain pasta, rinse, then toss with enough dressing to coat.
5. Add Parmesan cheese to pasta and refrigerate for at least 12 hours.
6. Add the remaining vegetables, herb seasoning blend, and paprika, and toss 2 hours before serving. Add more dressing if needed or desired.
7. Refrigerate until ready to serve.

Nutrition Facts Per Serving:

Calories: 260.52 kcal
Total Fat: 15.73 g
Cholesterol: 2 mg
Sodium: 32 mg
Carbohydrates: 27 g
Dietary Fiber: 2.2 g
Protein: 6 g
Potassium: 175 mg
Phosphorus: 77 mg

237. Picnic Potato Salad

Preparation Time: 15 minutes
Cooking Time: 10 minutes
Servings: 2

Ingredients:

- 3 eggs, large
- 1 stalk celery, finely chopped
- 1 medium potatoes
- 1 small onion, finely chopped
- 3/4 cup lite mayonnaise with olive oil
- 1/2 red bell pepper, finely chopped
- 1 teaspoon Dijon mustard
- 3 tablespoons cider vinegar
- 1/2 teaspoon black pepper

Directions:

1. Hard boil the eggs.
2. Set to boil the potatoes until tender but still firm when punctured with a fork. (To reduce potassium in potatoes, peel potatoes, cut into small pieces, cover with water and bring to a boil. Discard the water and add fresh water.)
3. Meanwhile, peel and chop hard-boiled eggs.
4. Strain cooked potatoes and place them in a bowl. Add vegetables and chopped eggs without stirring.
5. For salad dressing, mix mayonnaise, cider vinegar, black pepper, and Dijon mustard together. Add to potatoes and toss gently.
6. Cover and chill until ready to serve.

Nutrition Facts Per Serving:

Calories: 748.28 kcal

Total Fat: 65.47 g
Carbs: 29.26 g
Protein: 12.78 g
Sodium: 528.74 mg
Potassium: 720 mg
Phosphorus: 222 mg

238. Turkey Salad

Preparation Time: 15 minutes

Cooking Time: 15 minutes

Servings: 2

Ingredients:

- 4 ounces cooked, unsalted turkey breast, cubed
- 1 medium red apple, diced
- 1/3 cup diced celery
- 2 tablespoons + 2 teaspoons finely chopped onion
- 1 tablespoon + 1 teaspoon mayonnaise
- 2 teaspoons apple juice

Directions:

1. Add all ingredients into a medium bowl. Stir together until well mixed.
2. Chill until ready to serve.

Calories: 360 kcal
Sodium: 128 mg
Total Carbohydrate: 8 g
Protein: 17 g
Potassium: 296 mg
Phosphorus: 136 mg
Total Fat: 11 g
Cholesterol: 60 mg
Dietary Fiber: 1.9 g

239. Tuna Pasta Salad

Preparation Time: 15 minutes
Cooking Time: 15 minutes
Servings: 4

Ingredients:

- 1 cup cooked bow-tie pasta
- 2 tablespoons celery, chopped
- 1 tablespoon yellow bell pepper, chopped
- 1 tablespoon green onion, chopped
- 1/2 teaspoon lemon zest
- 2 tablespoons low-fat mayonnaise
- 2 tablespoons low-sodium Italian salad dressing
- 2 1/2 ounces canned low-sodium tuna in water

Directions:

1. Combine cooked pasta, bell pepper, celery, lemon zest, and onion in a mixing bowl.
2. Whisk together salad dressing and mayonnaise in a separate bowl.
3. Pour dressing over pasta mixture.
4. Add tuna to the pasta mixture.
5. Merge gently until all ingredients are moist and well blended.
6. Refrigerate for about 1 hour to let flavors blend.

Nutrition Facts Per Serving:

Calories: 520 kcal
Total Fat: 6 g
Cholesterol: 15 mg
Sodium: 370 mg

Carbohydrates: 21 g
Dietary Fiber: 1.3 g
Protein: 74 g
Potassium: 1300 mg
Phosphorus: 800 mg

240. Fruited Chicken Salad

Preparation Time: 15 minutes

Cooking Time: 10 minutes

Servings: 3

Ingredients:

- 1 cooked chicken breast, boneless and skinless
- 1/4 stalk celery, chopped
- 2 tablespoons onion, chopped
- 1/4 medium apple, chopped
- 1 tablespoon seedless red grapes
- 1 tablespoon seedless green grapes
- 2 tablespoons canned water chestnuts
- A pinch black pepper
- A pinch curry powders
- 3 tablespoons mayonnaise

Directions:

1. Dice chicken. Drain and chop water chestnuts.
2. Combine the chicken, onion, celery, apple, grapes, water chestnuts, pepper, curry powder, and mayonnaise in a large salad bowl and toss all together.
3. Serve immediately or chill for later.

Nutrition Facts Per Serving:

Calories 170Kcal
Total Fat: 18 g
Cholesterol: 44 mg
Sodium: 162 mg
Total Carbohydrate: 6 g
Dietary Fiber: 1.1 g
Protein: 14 g
Potassium: 200 mg
Phosphorus: 115 mg

241. Kidney-Friendly Cucumber Salad

Preparation Time: 15 minutes

Cooking Time: 10 minutes

Servings: 4

Ingredients:

- 1 medium cucumber, sliced (peeled or unpeeled)
- 1/4 medium onion, sliced
- 1/8 cup brown sugar
- 1/4 cup white vinegar
- 1/8 cup water
- A pinch salt (optional)

Directions:

1. In a bowl, combine cucumbers and onions. Sprinkle with salt. (Optional)
2. Boil vinegar, sugar, and water on medium-high heat until sugar is dissolved.
3. Pour vinegar mixture (while hot) over cucumbers. Mix well. Allow to sit before eating.

Nutrition Facts Per Serving:

Calories 70kcal
Total Fat: 0.2 g
Cholesterol: 0 mg
Sodium: 77.3 mg
Total Carbohydrate: 4.6 g
Dietary Fiber: 1.1 g
Protein: 0.8 g
Potassium: 191.8 mg
Phosphorus: 30 mg

242. Lettuce and Mushroom Salad

Preparation Time: 15 minutes

Cooking Time: 5 minutes

Servings: 2

Ingredients:

- 1 1/2 cups butter head lettuce
- 1/2 cup sliced mushrooms

- 2 tablespoons red onion, chopped
- 1/4 cup carrots, shredded

Directions:

1. Merge vegetables in a large bowl and toss. Serve in chilled salad bowls.

Nutrition Facts Per Serving:

Calories 30kcal
Total Fat: 0 g
Cholesterol: 0 mg
Total Carbohydrate: 4 g
Dietary Fiber: 1.2 g
Protein: 0 g
Sodium: 8 mg
Potassium: 230 mg
Phosphorus: 38 mg

243. Cranberries Spring Salad

Preparation Time: 15 minutes
Cooking Time: 0 minutes
Servings: 2

Ingredients:

- 1/2 cup of cooked lentils
- 1/2 cup of finely chopped arugula
- 1/2 cucumber, sliced
- 1/2 orange, peeled and sectioned
- 1/2 carrot, sliced
- 1/2 green bell pepper, sliced
- 1/4 cup of fresh cranberries
- 1/4 cup of olive oil
- 1/2 tsp. of ground red pepper
- 1/4 tsp. of salt
- 1 tsp. of balsamic vinegar

Directions:

1. Combine the vegetables in a large bowl. Add lentils and mix well. Set aside.
2. In a smaller bowl, shake together the balsamic vinegar, olive oil, salt, and red pepper. Put the vinaigrette over the vegetables and mix well. Top with orange and cranberries.
3. Serve cold.

Calories: 466.15 kcal

Total Fat: 29.32 g

Carbs: 41.15 g

Protein: 13.09 g

Sodium: 308.92 mg

Potassium: 590 mg

Phosphorus: 190 mg

244. Caesar Salad

Preparation Time: 5 minutes

Cooking Time: 5 minutes

Servings: 4

Ingredients:

- 1 head romaine lettuce
- 1/4 cup lite mayonnaise
- 1 tablespoon lemon juice
- 4 anchovy fillets
- 1 teaspoon Worcestershire sauce
- Black pepper
- 5 garlic cloves
- 4 tablespoons. cheddar cheese
- 1 teaspoon mustard

Directions:

1. In a bowl mix all ingredients and mix well
2. Serve with dressing

Nutrition Facts Per
Serving:

Calories: 186.34 kcal

Fat: 11.13 g

Sodium: 672.01 mg

Potassium: 800 mg

Carbs: 4.3 g

Protein: 3.2 g

Phosphorus: 160 mg

245. Summer Potato Salad

Preparation Time: 5 minutes

Cooking time: 0 minutes

Servings: 4

Ingredients:

- 2 1/4 cups potato, boiled, peeled and diced
- 3 tablespoons celery, chopped
- 3 tablespoons onion, chopped

- 3 tablespoons green pepper, chopped
- 2 chopped hard-boiled eggs, peeled and diced
- 1/4 cup lite mayonnaise
- 2 teaspoons vinegar
- 1/8 teaspoon dry mustard
- 1/8 teaspoon dried parsley
- 1/8 teaspoon paprika
- 1 pinch pepper
- 1 pinch garlic powder

Directions:

1. Take a suitable salad bowl.
2. Start tossing in all the ingredients.
3. Mix well and serve.

Nutrition Facts Per Serving:

Calories: 396.74 kcal
Total Fat: 26.11 g
Carbs: 32.58 g
Protein: 9.35 g
Sodium: 207.6 mg
Potassium: 820 mg
Phosphorus: 180 mg

246. Barb's Asian Slaw

Preparation Time: 5 minutes
Cooking Time: 5 minutes
Servings: 2

Ingredients:

- 1 small kale head, shredded
- 4 chopped green onions
- 1/2 cup slivered or sliced almonds
- Dressing:
- 1/2 cup olive oil
- 1/4 low-sodium soy sauce
- 1 tablespoon honey or maple syrup
- 1 tablespoon baking stevia

Directions:

1. Heat up dressing ingredients in a saucepan on the stove until thoroughly mixed.
2. Mix all ingredients when you are ready to serve.

Calories: 205kcal
Protein: 27g
Carbohydrate: 12g
Fat: 10 g
Calcium: 29 mg
Phosphorous: 76mg
Potassium: 27mg
Sodium: 111 mg

247. Italian Cucumber Salad

Preparation Time: 5 minutes

Cooking Time: 0 minutes

Servings: 2

Ingredients:

- 1/4 cup rice vinegar
- 1/8 teaspoon stevia
- 1/2 teaspoon olive oil
- 1/8 teaspoon black pepper
- 1/2 cucumber, sliced
- 1 cup carrots, sliced
- 2 tablespoons green onion, sliced
- 2 tablespoons red bell pepper, sliced
- 1/2 teaspoon Italian seasoning blend

Direction:

1. Put all the salad ingredients into a suitable salad bowl.
2. Toss them well and refrigerate for 1 hour.
3. Serve.

Nutrition Facts Per Serving:

Calories: 112 kcal
Total Fat 1.6 g
Cholesterol: 0 mg
Sodium: 43 mg
Protein: 2.3 g
Phosphorous: 198 mg
Potassium: 529 mg

248. Grapes Jicama Salad

Preparation Time: 5 minutes

Cooking Time: 0 minutes

Servings: 2

Ingredients:

- 1 cup jicama, peeled and sliced
- 1 carrot, sliced
- 1/2 medium red onion, sliced
- 1 1/4 cup seedless grapes
- 1/3 cup fresh basil leaves
- 1 tablespoon apple cider vinegar
- 1 1/2 tablespoon lemon juice
- 1 1/2 tablespoon lime juice

Direction:

1. Put all the salad ingredients into a suitable salad bowl.
2. Toss them well and refrigerate for 1 hour.
3. Serve.

Nutrition Facts Per Serving:

Calories 203
Total Fat 0.7g
Sodium: 44mg
Protein: 3.7 g
Calcium: 79 mg
Phosphorous: 141 mg
Potassium: 820 mg

249. Cucumber Couscous Salad

Preparation Time: 5 minutes

Cooking Time: 0 minutes

Servings: 4

Ingredients:

- 1 cucumber, sliced
- 1/2 cup red bell pepper, sliced
- 1/4 cup sweet onion, sliced
- 1/4 cup parsley, chopped
- 1/2 cup couscous, cooked
- 2 tablespoons olive oil
- 2 tablespoons rice vinegar
- 2 tablespoons feta cheese crumbled

274

- 1 1/2 teaspoon dried basil
- 1/4 teaspoon black pepper

Direction:

1. Put all the salad ingredients into a suitable salad bowl.
2. Toss them well and refrigerate for 1 hour.
3. Serve.

Nutrition Facts Per Serving:

Calories: 370 kcal
Total Fat: 9.8 g
Sodium: 258 mg
Protein: 6.2 g
Calcium: 80 mg
Phosphorous: 192 mg
Potassium: 209 mg

250. Carrot Jicama Salad

Preparation Time: 5 minutes

Cooking Time: 0 minutes

Servings: 2

Ingredients:

- 2 cup carrots, julienned
- 1 cup jicama, julienned
- 2 tablespoons lime juice
- 1 tablespoon olive oil
- 1/2 tablespoon apple cider
- 1/2 teaspoon brown Swerve

Direction:

1. Put all the salad ingredients into a suitable salad bowl.
2. Toss them well and refrigerate for 1 hour.
3. Serve.

Nutrition Facts Per Serving:

Calories: 173 kcal
Total Fat: 7.1 g
Sodium: 80 mg

Protein: 1.6 g

Calcium: 50 mg

Phosphorous: 96 mg

Potassium: 501 mg

251. Butterscotch Apple Salad

Preparation Time: 5 minutes

Cooking Time: 0 minutes

Servings: 6

Ingredients:

- 3 cups jazz apples, chopped
- 8 oz. canned crushed pineapple
- 8 oz. whipped topping
- 1/2 cup butterscotch topping
- 1/3 cup almonds
- 1/4 cup butterscotch

Direction:

1. Put all the salad ingredients into a suitable salad bowl.
2. Toss them well and refrigerate for 1 hour.
3. Serve.

Calories: 293 kcal

Total Fat: 12.7 g

Sodium: 52 mg

Protein: 4.2 g

Calcium: 65 mg

Phosphorous: 202 mg

Potassium: 296 mg

252. Cranberry Cabbage Slaw

Preparation Time: 5 minutes

Cooking Time: 0 minutes

Servings: 4

Ingredients:

- 1/2 medium cabbage head, shredded
- 1 medium red apple, shredded
- 2 tablespoons onion, sliced
- 1/2 cup dried cranberries
- 1/4 cup almonds, toasted sliced
- 1/2 cup olive oil
- 1/4 teaspoon stevia

- 1/4 cup cider vinegar
- 1/2 tablespoon celery seed
- 1/2 teaspoon dry mustard
- 1/2 cup lite or 40% fat cream

Direction:

1. Take a suitable salad bowl.
2. Start tossing in all the ingredients.
3. Mix well and serve.

Nutrition Facts Per Serving:

Calories: 823.13 kcal
Total Fat: 63.95 g
Carbs: 65.89 g
Sugars: 48.19 g
Protein: 6.46 g
Sodium: 57.31 mg
Potassium: 711 mg
Phosphorus: 114 mg

253. Chestnut Noodle Salad

Preparation Time: 5 minutes
Cooking Time: 0 minutes
Servings: 6

Ingredients:

- 8 cups cabbage, shredded
- 1/2 cup canned chestnuts, sliced
- 6 green onions, chopped
- 1/4 cup olive oil
- 1/4 cup apple cider vinegar
- 3/4 teaspoon stevia
- 1/8 teaspoon black pepper
- 1 cup chow Mein noodles, cooked

Direction:

1. Take a suitable salad bowl.
2. Start tossing in all the ingredients.
3. Mix well and serve.

Calories: 390 kcal

Total Fat: 13 g

Cholesterol: 1 mg

Sodium: 78 mg

Protein: 4.2 g

Calcium: 142 mg

Phosphorous: 188 mg

Potassium: 302 mg

254. Pineapple Berry Salad

Preparation Time: 5 minutes

Cooking time: 0 minutes

Servings: 4

Ingredients:

- 3 cups pineapple, peeled and cubed
- 3 cups strawberries, chopped
- 1/4 cup honey
- 1/2 cup basil leaves
- 1 tablespoon lemon zest
- 1/2 cup blueberries

Directions:

1. Take a suitable salad bowl.
2. Start tossing in all the ingredients.
3. Mix well and serve.

Nutrition Facts Per Serving:

Calories: 349.19 kcal

Total Fat: 1.16 g

Cholesterol: 0 mg

Sodium: 7.25 mg

Carbohydrate: 90.81 g

Sugars: 23.4 g

Protein: 1.8 g

Phosphorous: 85 mg

Potassium: 620 mg

255. Thai Cucumber Salad

Preparation Time: 5 minutes

Cooking Time: 5 minutes

Servings: 2

Ingredients:

- 1/4 cup chopped peanuts
- 1/4 cup brown sugar

- 1/2 cup cilantro
- 1/4 cup rice wine vinegar
- 3 cucumbers
- 2 jalapeno peppers

Directions:

1. Mix all the ingredients in a bowl.
2. Serve with dressing

Nutrition Facts Per Serving:

Calories: 20 kcal
Fat: 0 g
Sodium: 85 mg
Carbs: 5 g
Protein: 1 g
Potassium: 190.4 mg
Phosphorus: 46.8 mg

256. Red Potato Salad

Preparation Time: 5 minutes

Cooking Time: 5 minutes

Servings: 2

Ingredients:

- 2 cups of mayonnaise
- 0.25 pound of bacon
- 1 stalk celery
- 4 eggs
- Pepper
- 1 red sweet potato
- 1 onion

Directions:

1. In a pot, add water, potatoes, and cook until tender.
2. Remove, drain, and set aside.
3. Place eggs in a saucepan, add water and bring to a boil.
4. Cover and let eggs stand for 10–15 minutes.
5. When ready, remove, meanwhile in a deep skillet, cook bacon on low heat.
6. Slice celery and onion in wings, Mix all the ingredients in a bowl.
7. Serve with dressing.

Nutrition Facts Per Serving:

Calories: 424.61 kcal
Total Fat: 29.17 g
Carbs: 23.98 g

Protein: 17.02 g

Sodium: 394.27 mg

Potassium: 700 mg

Phosphorus: 300 mg

257. Broccoli-Cauliflower Salad

Preparation Time: 5 minutes

Cooking Time: 5 minutes

Servings: 4

Ingredients:

- 1 tbsp. of wine vinegar
- 1 cup of cauliflower florets
- 1/4 cup of white sugar
- 2 hard-cooked eggs
- 3 slices of bacon
- 1 cup of broccoli florets
- 1 cup of cheddar cheese
- 1tbsp of lite mayonnaise

Directions:

1. Boil the cauliflower florets for 5 minutes.
2. Mix all the ingredients in a bowl.
3. Serve with dressing.

Nutrition Facts Per Serving:

Calories: 219.3 kcal

Total Fat: 19.07 g

Protein: 10.26 g

Sodium: 310.73 mg

Potassium: 134 mg

Phosphorus: 141 mg

258. Macaroni Salad

Preparation Time: 5 minutes

Cooking Time: 0 minute

Servings: 4

Ingredients:

- 1/4 tsp. of celery seed
- 2 hard-boiled eggs
- 2 cups of salad dressing
- 1 sliced onion
- 2 tsps. white vinegar
- 2 stalks of celery
- 2 cups of cooked macaroni
- 1 red bell pepper
- 2 tbsps. of mustard

1. Mix all the ingredients in a bowl.
2. Serve with dressing.

Nutrition Facts Per Serving:

Calories: 360 kcal
Fat: 21 g
Sodium: 400 mg
Carbs: 36 g
Protein: 6 g
Potassium: 68 mg
Phosphorus: 36 mg

259. Green Bean and Potato Salad

Preparation Time: 5 minutes
Cooking Time: 5 minutes
Servings: 4

Ingredients:

- 1/2 cup of basil
- 1/4 cup of olive oil
- 1 tbsp. of mustard
- 3/4 lb. of green beans
- 1 tbsp. of lemon juice
- 1/2 cup of balsamic vinegar
- 1 red onion
- 1 lb. of red potatoes
- 1 garlic clove

Directions:

1. Boil potatoes using a pot for 15–18 minutes or until tender.
2. Throw in the green beans after 5–6 minutes.
3. Drain and cut into cubes.
4. In a bowl, attach all ingredients and mix well.
5. Serve with dressing.

Nutrition Facts Per Serving:

Calories: 153.2 kcal
Fat: 2.0 g
Sodium: 77.6 mg
Potassium: 759.0 mg
Carbs: 29.0 g
Protein: 6.9 g
Phosphorus: 49 mg

260. Spinach Salad with Orange Vinaigrette

Preparation Time: 10 minutes

Cooking Time: 0 minute

Servings: 4

Ingredients:

1. Zest and juice of 1 mandarin orange
2. 1 tablespoon of extra-virgin olive oil
3. Freshly ground black pepper
4. 6 ounces of baby spinach
5. 2 mandarin oranges, peeled, membranes removed

Directions:

1. In a small bowl, whip the orange zest, orange juice, and olive oil. Season with pepper.
2. In a medium bowl, blend the spinach and pieces of orange. Drizzle the dressing over the salad, and toss to coat.
3. Serve and enjoy!

Nutrition Facts Per Serving:

Calories: 73 kcal

Total fat: 4 g

Cholesterol: 0 mg

Carbohydrates: 10 g

Protein: 2 g

Phosphorus 33 mg

Potassium: 353 mg

Sodium: 35 mg

261. Mixed Green Leaf and Citrus Salad

Preparation Time: 10 minutes

Cooking Time: 0 minute

Servings: 4

Ingredients:

- 4 cups of mixed salad greens
- Juice of 1 lemon
- 2 teaspoons of extra-virgin olive oil
- Freshly ground black pepper

282

- 1 orange, peeled and thinly sliced
- 1/2 lemon, peeled and thinly sliced
- 4 tablespoons of (1/4 cup) dried cranberries
- 4 tablespoons of (1/4 cup) pitted Kalamata olives

Directions:

1. In a large bowl, blend the greens, lemon juice, and olive oil. Flavor with pepper.
2. Set the greens on four plates, and top each with 2 slices of orange and lemon.
3. Attach 1 tablespoon each of cranberries and Kalamata olives to each plate.
4. Serve.

Nutrition Facts Per Serving:

Calories: 193 kcal
Total fat: 9 g
Cholesterol: 0 mg
Carbohydrates: 15 g
Fiber: 2 g
Phosphorus: 116 mg
Potassium: 219 mg
Sodium: 137 mg

262. Roasted Beet Salad

Preparation Time: 10 minutes

Cooking Time: 30 minutes

Servings: 4

Ingredients:

- 6 beets, trimmed
- 2 tablespoons of plus 1 teaspoon extra-virgin olive oil, divided
- 1 tablespoon of white wine vinegar
- 1 teaspoon of Dijon mustard
- Freshly ground black pepper
- 2 cups of baby salad greens
- 1/2 sweet onion, sliced
- 2 tablespoons of crumbled feta cheese
- 2 tablespoons of walnut pieces

283

Directions:

1. Preheat the oven to 400F.
2. Blend the beets with 1 teaspoon of olive oil, wrap them in aluminum foil, and cook for 30 minutes, until fork-tender.
3. In a small bowl, merge the remaining 2 tablespoons of olive oil, vinegar, and mustard—season with pepper.
4. In a medium bowl, mix the salad greens, onion, feta cheese, and walnuts. Toss with about half of the vinaigrette. Arrange on four plates.
5. Slice the beets into wedges and top the salads. Serve with the remaining dressing.

Nutrition Facts Per Serving:

Calories: 270kcal
Total fat: 39g
Cholesterol: 4mg
Carbohydrates: 20g
Phosphorus 93 mg

Potassium: 58 5mg
Sodium: 217 mg

263. Pesto Pasta Salad

Preparation Time: 15 minutes
Cooking Time: 25 minutes
Servings: 4

Ingredients:

- 1 cup fresh basil leaves
- 1/2 cup packed parsley leaves
- 1/2 cup arugula, chopped
- 2 tbsps. cheddar cheese, grated
- 3 tbsp. extra-virgin olive oil
- 3 tbsps. lite mayonnaise
- 2 tbsps. water
- 4 oz. whole wheat rotini pasta
- 1 red bell pepper, chopped
- 1 medium yellow summer squash, sliced
- 1 cup baby peas, frozen

Directions:

1. Take a large pot and boil water.
2. Meanwhile, take a blender (or a food processor) and combine the basil, parsley, arugula, cheese, and olive oil.
3. Process until the herbs are finely chopped. Add the mayonnaise and water, and then process again. Set aside.
4. Now, put the pasta into the pot with boiling water, and cook according to package directions, about 12 minutes. Drain well, reserving 1/4 cup of the cooking liquid.
5. Mix the pesto, pasta, bell pepper, squash, and peas in a large bowl and toss gently, adding enough reserved pasta cooking liquid to make a sauce on the salad.
6. Serve immediately or cover and chill, then serve.

7. Cover and store it in the refrigerator for up to 3 days.

Nutrition Facts Per Serving:

Calories: 450kcal
Fats: 24 g
Carbs: 35 g
Protein: 9 g
Sodium: 163 mg
Potassium: 472 mg
Phosphorus: 213 mg

264. Appealing Green Salad

Preparation Time: 10 minutes

Cooking Time: 0 minutes

Servings: 4

Ingredients:

For Dressing:

- 1 tbsp. of shallot, minced
- 2 tbsp. of olive oil
- 2 tbsp. of fresh lemon juice
- 1 tsp. of honey

285

- Freshly ground black pepper, to taste

For Salad:

- 1 1/2 cups of chopped broccoli florets
- 1 1/2 cups of shredded cabbage
- 4 cups of chopped lettuce

Directions:

1. In a bowl, add all dressing ingredients and beat till well combined. Keep aside.
2. In another large bowl, mix all salad ingredients.
3. Add dressing and gently toss to coat well.
4. Serve immediately.

Nutrition Facts Per Serving:

Calories: 179 kcal
Fat: 17.1g
Carbs: 7.5 g
Protein: 1.7 g
Fiber: 1.9 g
Potassium: 249 mg
Sodium: 21 mg

265. Mango with Avocado Salad

Preparation Time: 10 minutes
Cooking Time: 0 minute
Servings: 4

Ingredients:

- 1 chopped Lettuce
- 1 pinch of Pepper
- 1 Avocado
- 1 Mango
- 1 tablespoon of White wine vinegar
- 1 tablespoon of olive oil
- 2 tablespoons of chopped toasted almonds
- 2 tablespoons of dried cranberries

Directions:

1. Peel and chop the vegetables.
2. Put the lettuce, mango, avocado, almonds, and cranberries in a bowl.
3. On the other hand, mix the oil with the vinegar and add pepper for dressing.

4. Pour over the salad and mix.
5. Serve on plates and enjoy.

Nutrition Facts Per Serving:

Calories: 34 kcal
Carbohydrates: 19.59 g
Proteins: 4.15 g
Fiber: 5.77 g
Fat: 22 g
Sodium: 57 mg

266. Avocado and Lettuce Salad

Preparation Time: 10 minutes
Cooking Time: 0 minute
Servings: 2

Ingredients:

- 1 tomato
- 1 lettuce
- 1/2 red pepper, diced julienne
- 1 pinch of Pepper
- 1 Avocado
- 2 tablespoons of Nuez chopped (walnut crepes)
- 2 tablespoon of Modena balsamic vinegar
- 2 tablespoon of lemon juice
- 1 pinch of extra virgin olive oil

Directions:

1. Wash the lettuce well and chop it.
2. Wash and chop the remaining ingredients such as the Tomato, red pepper or diced julienne, Avocado, Nuez chopped Modena balsamic vinegar.
3. Mix the lemon juice, vinegar, virgin oil, and pepper. Then toss on the salad.
4. Remove and add the nuts (optional) to garnish.

Nutrition Facts Per Serving:

Calories: 315.5 kcal
Carbohydrates: 10.8 g
Proteins: 6.55 g
Fiber: 7.55 g
Fat: 25.88 g
Sodium: 120 mg
Potassium: 730 mg

267. Rocket Salad with Mango, Avocado, and Cherry Tomatoes

Preparation Time: 10 minutes

Cooking Time: 0 minute

Servings: 2

Ingredients:

- 1 tbsp. of lime juice
- 2 tbsps. of white balsamic vinegar
- 2 tbsps. of rapeseed oil
- 2 tbsps. of olive oil
- 1 tsp. of honey
- 1 tsp. of medium-hot mustard
- Pepper
- 3 handful of rockets (120g)
- 200g of cherry tomatoes
- 1/2 ripe mango
- 1 avocado

Directions:

1. For the vinaigrette, whip lime juice with balsamic vinegar, rapeseed, and olive oils.
2. Whisk in honey and mustard and then season with pepper.
3. Wash the rocket and spin dry.
4. Wash tomatoes and halve.
5. Peel the mango, slice the pulp from the core, and dice it.
6. Halve the avocado, core it, remove the pulp from the skin and dice it as well.
7. Add cherry tomatoes, ripe mango, avocado
8. Pour all the salad ingredients inside a bowl with the vinaigrette, and spread on four plates.

Nutrition Facts Per Serving:

Calories: 455.52 kcal

Total Fat: 39.37 g

Carbs: 27.47 g

Sugars: 18.65 g

Sodium: 40.1 mg

Potassium: 720 mg

Phosphorus: 72 mg

268. Chickpea Salad

Preparation Time: 5 minutes

Cooking Time: 10 minutes

Servings: 2

Ingredients:

- 1 garlic (one clove)
- ½ cup of chickpeas
- 1 onion, medium
- 1 red pepper
- Pinch of paprika
- Pinch of pepper
- Parsley (one bunch)
- 1 pinch of salt (optional)
- 2 tbsp. of vinegar
- 2 tbsp. of olive oil
- 1 unit (s) of green pepper
- 200 grams of canned garbanzo
- 1 tablespoon of lemon juice

Directions:

1. Chop all the red peppers, Green pepper, onion, and parsley and mix them with the chickpeas.
2. In a separate bowl, mix an abundant stream of oil, another stream of vinegar, lemon juice, a teaspoon of paprika (sweet), a pinch of pepper, a clove of garlic, chopped into small pieces, and a little salt (optional).
3. Add the canned Garbanzo
4. Then add the dressing to the vegetables.

Nutrition Facts Per Serving:

Calories: 511.42kcal

Carbohydrates: 37.33g

Proteins: 16.66g

Fiber: 15 g

Fat: 19 g

Sodium: 330 mg

Potassium: 900 mg

Phosphorus: 340 mg

269. Bulgur and Broccoli Salad

Preparation Time: 10 minutes

Cooking Time: 15 minutes

Servings: 4

Ingredients:

- 3 cups of broccoli florets
- 1 cup of bulgur
- 1/2 cup of halved cherry tomatoes
- 1/4 cup of raw sunflower seeds
- 1/4 cup of chopped mint leaves
- Juice of 1 lemon
- 1 tablespoon of extra-virgin olive oil

Directions:

1. In a medium bowl, prepare an ice-water bath by filling the bowl with ice and water.
2. Set the water to boil. Attach the broccoli and blanch for 3 minutes.
3. With a slotted spoon, remove the broccoli and transfer it to the ice bath, retaining the cooking water over the heat.
4. Once cool, after about 3 minutes, drain the ice and water. Set the broccoli aside.
5. Add the bulgur to the hot water; remove from the heat, cover, and let sit for 15 minutes.
6. Drain, pressing the bulgur with the back of a spoon to remove excess moisture.
7. In a medium bowl, toss the broccoli, bulgur, tomatoes, sunflower seeds, mint, lemon juice, and olive oil.
8. Serve immediately.

Nutrition Facts Per Serving:

Calories: 250 kcal

Fat: 6 g

Carbs: 24 g

Protein: 6 g

Phosphorus: 101 mg

Potassium: 315 mg

Sodium: 21 mg

270. Pear and Watercress Salad

Preparation Time: 10 minutes

Cooking Time: 0 minute

Servings: 4

Ingredients:

- 1/4 cup of sweet onion, coarsely chopped
- 1 teaspoon of Dijon mustard
- 2 tablespoons of extra-virgin olive oil
- 1 tablespoon of white wine vinegar
- 1 teaspoon of honey
- 1 bunch of watercress, thick stems removed, washed well
- 2 ripe pears
- 0.5 lb. of crumbled feta cheese

Directions:

1. In a food processor or blender, merge the onion, mustard, olive oil, vinegar, and honey.
2. Process until smooth.
3. In a medium bowl, blend the watercress with the dressing.
4. Arrange on four plates.
5. Top each with pear slices and crumbled feta cheese.

Nutrition Facts Per Serving:

Calories: 144 kcal

Fat: 8g

Carbs: 17g

Protein: 3g

Phosphorus: 70mg

Potassium: 310 mg

Sodium: 134 mg

271. Tropical Chicken Salad

Preparation Time: 20 minutes

Cooking Time: 0 minute

Servings: 4

Ingredients:

- 1/2 cup of diced celery
- 1 1/2 cup of shredded cooked chicken
- 1 cup of peeled and diced apples

- 1 cup of drained unsweetened pineapple chunks
- 1/2 cup of seedless grapes
- 1 cup of diced pears
- 2 tbsp. of lemon juice
- 2 tbsp. of lite mayonnaise
- Dash hot sauce
- 1 tsp. of pepper
- Paprika for garnish

Directions:

1. Mix juice, mayo, hot sauce, and pepper.
2. In a large bowl, merge together the rest of the ingredients.
3. Add dressing to fruit and chicken and combine well.
4. Serve with paprika.

Nutrition Facts Per Serving:

Calories: 443.8
Fat: 25 g
Protein: 33.1 g
Sodium: 150 mg
Phosphorus: 170 mg
Potassium: 563.5 mg

272. Chicken and Grape Salad

Preparation Time: 20 minutes
Cooking Time: 0 minute
Servings: 6

Ingredients:

- 1 diced apple
- 1 cup of rotelle pasta cooked (according to package directions)
- 1/2 cup of seedless grapes
- 1 half breast of sliced cooked chicken

Dressing:
- 2 tbsp. of lite mayonnaise
- 2 tbsp. of sriracha hot sauce
- 1/4 cup of light sour cream

Directions:

1. Merge dressing ingredients in a large bowl and mix well.
2. Add cooked pasta and mix well.
3. Add grapes and apples and mix well.

4. Set to serving plates and top with sliced chicken.

Nutrition Facts Per Serving:

Calories: 558.71 kcal
Total Fat: 21.67 g
Carbs: 51.45 g
Protein: 38.87 g
Sodium: 657.34 mg
Potassium: 620 mg
Phosphorus: 300 mg

273. Fresh Berry Salad

Preparation Time: 15 minutes
Cooking Time: 0 minute
Servings: 4

Ingredients:

- 3 tbsp. of balsamic vinegar
- 2 tbsp. of honey
- Dash of ground cardamom
- Ground pepper
- ½ cup of hulled and quartered strawberries
- ½ cup of blueberries
- 1 sprig mint leaves roughly torn

Directions:

1. Whip together in a large bowl the vinegar, honey, pepper, and cardamom.
2. Tumble in the berries and mint leaves.
3. Serve chilled.

Nutrition Facts Per Serving:

Calories: 120 kcal
Carbs: 30 g
Sugars: 28 g
Protein: 1 g
Sodium: 51.5 mg
Phosphorus: 3.7 mg
Potassium: 394 mg

274. Almond Pasta Salad

Cooking time: 0 minutes
Servings: 14

Ingredients:

- 1cup elbow macaroni, cooked

- 1/2 cup sun-dried tomatoes, diced
- 1 (15 oz.) can whole artichokes, diced
- 1 orange bell pepper, diced
- 3 green onions, sliced
- 2 tablespoons basil, sliced
- 2 oz. slivered almonds

Dressing:
- 1 garlic clove, minced
- 1 tablespoon Dijon mustard
- 1 tablespoon raw honey
- 1/4 cup white balsamic vinegar
- 2 tbsp. olive oil

Directions:

1. Take a suitable salad bowl.
2. Start tossing in all the ingredients.
3. Mix well and serve.

Nutrition Facts Per Serving:

Calories: 444.29 kcal
Total Fat: 15.58 g
Carbs: 65.19 g

Protein: 19.01 g
Sodium: 153.75 mg
Potassium: 1000 mg
Phosphorus: 300 mg

275. Tofu and Rice Salad Bowl

Preparation time: 20 minutes

Cooking time: 40 minutes

Servings: 4

Ingredients:

For the Dressing
- 2 tablespoons apple cider vinegar
- 2 garlic cloves, minced
- 2 tablespoons extra-virgin olive oil
- 1 tablespoon tahini
- 1/4 cup water

For the Salad
- 1 (14-ounce) package extra-firm tofu
- 1 tablespoon sesame oil
- 1 cup white rice
- 4 cups mixed salad greens
- 1 beet, peeled and grated
- 2 carrots, grated

294

- 1/4 cup sunflower seeds

Directions:

To Make the Dressing

1. In a small bowl, merge the vinegar, garlic, olive oil, tahini, and water. Set aside.

To Make the Salad

1. Preheat the oven to 350F. Line a baking sheet with parchment paper.
2. Cut the tofu into bite-size rectangles about 1/2 inch thick. Pour with the sesame oil, and arrange in a single layer on the prepared baking sheet. Bake for 15 minutes.
3. Prepare the rice according to package directions, for about 20 minutes.
4. Place a scoop of rice in each of four bowls, and then top each with 1 cup of salad greens and equal portions of the beet, carrots, and sunflower seeds. Top with the baked tofu and serve with the dressing.

Nutrition Facts Per Serving:

Calories: 563.36 kcal
Total Fat: 27.39 g
Carbs: 55.19 g
Protein: 27.02 g
Sodium: 120.01 mg
Potassium: 640 mg
Phosphorus: 230 mg

Vegetables

276. Chili Tofu Noodles

> **Preparation time: 5 minutes**
> **Cooking time: 50 minutes**
> **Servings: 4**

Ingredients:

- 1/2 diced red chili
- 1 cup rice noodles
- 1/2 juiced lime
- 6 ounces pressed and cubed silken firm tofu
- 1 teaspoon grated fresh ginger
- 1 tablespoon coconut oil
- 1 cup green beans
- 1 minced garlic clove

Directions:

1. Steam the green beans for 10-12 minutes or according to package directions and drain.
2. Cook the noodles in a pot of boiling water for 10-15 minutes or according to package directions.
3. Meanwhile, heat a wok or skillet on a high heat and add coconut oil.
4. Now add the tofu, chili flakes, garlic and ginger and sauté for 5-10 minutes.
5. After doing that, drain in the noodles along with the green beans and lime juice then add it to the wok.
6. Toss to coat.
7. Serve hot!

Nutrition Facts Per Serving:

Calories 313 kcal
Protein: 10 g
Carbs: 28 g
Fat: 12 g
Sodium: 99 mg
Potassium: 312 mg
Phosphorus: 120 mg

277. Curried Cauliflower

Preparation time: 5 minutes

Cooking time: 25 minutes

Servings: 4

Ingredients:

- 1 teaspoon turmeric
- 1 diced onion
- 1 tablespoon chopped fresh cilantro
- 1 teaspoon cumin
- 1/2 diced chili
- 1/2 cup water
- 1 minced garlic clove
- 1 tablespoon coconut oil
- 1 teaspoon garam masala
- 2 cups cauliflower florets

Directions:

1. Attach the oil to a skillet on medium heat.
2. Sauté the onion and garlic for 5 minutes until soft.
3. Add in the cumin, turmeric and garam masala and stir to release the aromas.
4. Now add the chili to the pan along with the cauliflower.
5. Stir to coat.
6. Pour in the water and reduce the heat to a simmer for 15 minutes.
7. Garnish with cilantro to serve.

Nutrition Facts Per Serving:

Calories: 133 kcal

Protein: 2 g

Carbs: 11 g

Fat: 7 g

Sodium: 35 mg

Potassium: 328 mg

Phosphorus: 39 mg

278. Elegant Veggie Tortillas

Preparation time: 30 minutes

Cooking time: 30 minutes

Servings: 12

Ingredients:

- 1/2 cup of chopped broccoli florets

- 1 1/2 cups of chopped cauliflower florets
- 1 tablespoon of water
- 2 teaspoon of canola oil
- 1 1/2 cups of chopped onion
- 1 minced garlic clove
- 2 tablespoons of finely chopped fresh parsley
- 1/2 cup of low-cholesterol liquid egg substitute
- Freshly ground black pepper, to taste
- 4 (6-inches) warmed corn tortillas

Directions:

1. In a microwave bowl, place broccoli, cauliflower and water and microwave, covered for about 3-5 minutes.
2. Remove from the microwave and drain any liquid.
3. Heat oil on medium heat.
4. Add onion and sauté for about 4-5 minutes.
5. Add garlic and then sauté it for about 1 minute.
6. Stir in broccoli, cauliflower, parsley, egg substitute and black pepper.
7. Reduce the heat and let it simmer for about 10 minutes.
8. Detach from heat and keep aside to cool slightly.
9. Place broccoli mixture over 1/4 of each tortilla.
10. Fold the outside edges inward and roll up like a burrito.
11. Secure each tortilla with toothpicks to secure the filling.
12. Cut each tortilla in half and serve.

Nutrition Facts Per Serving:

Calories: 539.19 kcal
Fat: 11.86 g
Carbs: 96.49 g
Protein: 8.1 g
Fiber: 6.3 g
Potassium: 950 mg
Sodium: 219.29 mg
Phosphorus: 600 mg

279. Simple Broccoli Stir-fry

Preparation time: 40 minutes

Cooking time: 15 minutes

Servings: 4

Ingredients:

- 1 tablespoon of olive oil
- 1 minced garlic clove
- 2 cups of broccoli florets
- 2 tablespoons of water

Directions:

1. Heat oil on medium heat.
2. Add garlic and then sauté for about 1 minute.
3. Attach the broccoli and stir fry for about 2 minutes.
4. Stir in water and stir fry for about 4-5 minutes.
5. Serve warm.

Nutrition Facts Per Serving:

Calories: 89 kcal

Fat: 3.6 g

Carbs: 3.3 g

Protein: 1.3 g

Fiber: 1.2 g

Potassium: 230 mg

Sodium: 23 mg

Phosphorus: 49 mg

280. Braised Cabbage

Preparation time: 30 minutes

Cooking time: 40 minutes

Servings: 4

Ingredients:

- 1 1/2 teaspoon of olive oil
- 2 minced garlic cloves
- 1 thinly sliced onion
- 3 cups of chopped green cabbage
- 1 cup of low-sodium vegetable broth
- Freshly ground black pepper, to taste

Directions:

1. In a large skillet, warm oil on medium-high heat.
2. Add garlic and then sauté for about 1 minute.

3. Add onion and sauté for about 4-5 minutes.
4. Add cabbage and sauté for about 3-4 minutes.
5. Stir in broth and black pepper and immediately, reduce the heat to low.
6. Cook, covered for about 20 minutes
7. Serve warm.

Nutrition Facts Per Serving:

Calories: 99 kcal
Fat: 1.8 g
Carbs: 6.6 g
Protein: 1.1 g
Fiber: 1.9 g
Potassium: 600 mg
Sodium: 99 mg
Phosphorus: 39 mg

281. Sautéed Green Beans

Preparation Time: 10 minutes
Cooking Time: 30 minutes
Servings: 4

Ingredients:

- 2 cup frozen green beans
- 1/2 cup red bell pepper
- 2 tsp. margarine
- 1/4 cup onion
- 1 tsp. dried dill weed
- 1 tsp. dried parsley
- 1/4 tsp. black pepper

Directions:

1. Cook green beans in a large pan of boiling water until tender, then drain.
2. While the beans are cooking, melt the margarine in a skillet and fry the other vegetables.
3. Add the beans to sautéed vegetables.
4. Sprinkle with freshly ground pepper and serve with meat and fish dishes.

Nutrition Facts Per Serving:

Calories: 130 kcal

Fat: 7 g

Carbs: 8 g

Protein: 4 g

Sodium: 76 mg

Potassium: 340 mg

Phosphorus: 55 mg

282. Penne Pasta with Asparagus

Preparation Time: 30 minutes

Cooking Time: 10 minutes

Servings: 4

Ingredients:

- 2 tbsp. unsalted butter
- 1 clove of garlic
- 1 tsp. red pepper
- 1 tsp. black pepper
- 1cup asparagus, cut into 2-inch pieces
- 2 tsp. lemon juice
- 4 cup whole wheat penne pasta, cooked
- 1/4 cup shredded cheddar cheese
- 1/4 tsp. Tabasco hot sauce

Directions:

1. Add unsalted butter in a skillet over medium heat.
2. Fry garlic and red pepper flakes for 2-3 minutes.
3. Add asparagus, Tabasco sauce, lemon juice, and black pepper to skillet and cook for a further 6 minutes.
4. Add pre-cooked, hot pasta and cheese. Toss and serve.

Nutrition Facts Per Serving:

Calories: 387 kcal

Carbs: 49 g

Protein: 13 g

Sodium: 93 mg

Potassium: 258 mg

Phosphorous: 252 mg

283. Garlic Mashed Potatoes

Preparation Time: 5 minutes
Cooking Time: 25 minutes
Servings: 4

Ingredients:

- 2 medium potatoes, peeled and sliced
- 2 tbsp. unsalted butter
- 1/4 cup 1% low-fat milk
- 2 garlic cloves

Directions:

1. Double-boil or soak the potatoes to reduce potassium if you are on a low potassium diet.
2. Boil potatoes and garlic until soft for about 20 minutes. Drain.
3. Beat the potatoes and garlic with butter and milk until smooth.

Nutrition Facts Per Serving:

Calories: 168 kcal
Fat: 12g
Carbs: 29 g
Protein: 5 g
Sodium: 59 mg
Potassium: 189 mg
Phosphorous: 57 mg

284. Cauliflower and Potato Curry

Preparation time: 40 minutes
Cooking time: 30minutes
Servings: 4

Ingredients:

- 2 tablespoons canola oil
- 1/2 sweet onion, chopped
- 2-inch piece ginger
- 3 garlic cloves, minced
- 1 teaspoon ground turmeric
- 1 teaspoon ground cumin
- 1 small head cauliflower, cut into florets
- 1 medium potato, diced
- 2 small tomatoes, diced
- 1 small green Chile, stemmed, seeded, and diced
- 1/2 cup water

- Juice of 1/2 lemon
- 1/4 cup chopped cilantro leaves
- 1 teaspoon garam masala
- ½ cup basmati rice or 1 whole wheat bread, for serving

Directions:

1. Warm up the olive oil. Add the onion and cook.
2. Attach the ginger and garlic, and cook until fragrant. Stir in the turmeric and cumin. Add the cauliflower, potato, tomatoes, Chile, and water. Bring to a simmer, reduce the heat, and cover.
3. Cook, stirring occasionally, for 25 minutes, until the potatoes and cauliflower are tender.
4. Stir in the lemon juice, cilantro, and garam masala. Serve over rice or with bread.

285. White Bean Veggie Burgers

Preparation time: 10 minutes
Cooking time: 25 minutes
Servings: 4

Ingredients:

- 1 cup canned white beans
- 1 cup cooked rice
- 1 teaspoon garlic powder
- 2 teaspoons dried thyme
- 1/2 teaspoon ground chipotle pepper
- 1/2 sweet onion, finely chopped

- 1/2 cup fresh or frozen corn
- 1/2 cup bell pepper
- Juice of 1 lemon
- 1/3 cup all-purpose flour
- 1 large egg
- Freshly ground black pepper
- 2 teaspoons extra-virgin olive oil

Directions:

1. In a large bowl, break the beans with a potato masher, leaving a few whole beans as desired. Attach the rice, garlic powder, thyme, chipotle pepper, onion, corn, bell pepper, lemon, flour, and egg, and merge well to blend. Sprinkle it with pepper.
2. With your hands, make the mixture into four patties.
3. In a skillet over medium heat, warm up the olive oil. Grill each burger. Serve.

Calories: 401.27 kcal
Total Fat: 8.37 g
Carbs: 67.88 g
Protein: 16.33 g
Sodium: 410.43 mg
Potassium: 800 mg
Phosphorus: 240 mg

286. Spinach Falafel Wrap

Preparation time: 10 minutes
Cooking time: 15 minutes
Servings: 4

Ingredients:

- 6 ounces baby spinach
- 1 (15-ounce) can chickpeas, drained and rinsed
- 2 teaspoons ground cumin
- 3/4 cup flour
- 2 tablespoons canola oil, divided, for frying
- 1/4 cup plain, unsweetened yogurt

305

- 2 garlic cloves, minced
- Juice of 1 lemon
- Freshly ground black pepper
- 4 tortillas
- 1 cucumber, cut into spears
- 2 slices red onion
- Salad greens, for serving

Directions:

1. Set the spinach in a colander in the sink, and pour boiling water over it to wilt the spinach. Allow it to cool.
2. In a food processor, attach the spinach, chickpeas, cumin, and flour. Pulse until just blended.
3. Divide the mixture into tablespoon-size balls, and use your hands to press them flat into patties.
4. In a large skillet over medium-high heat, warm up 1 tablespoon of oil. Add half of the falafel patties, and cook for 2 to 3 minutes on each side, until browned and crisp. Repeat with the remaining falafel patties.
5. In a small bowl, combine the yogurt, garlic, lemon juice, and pepper.
6. On each tortilla, place 3 falafel patties, a couple cucumber spears, a few red-onion rings, and a handful of salad greens. Set each with 1 tablespoon of the yogurt sauce.

Nutrition Facts Per Serving:

Calories: 687.45 kcal
Total Fat: 21.76 g
Carbs: 108.63 g
Protein: 21.06 g
Sodium: 461.27 mg
Potassium: 900 mg
Phosphorus: 600 mg

287. Spicy Tofu and Broccoli Stir-fry

Preparation time: 15 minutes

Cooking time: 30 minutes

Servings: 4

Ingredients:

For the Sauce
- 3 garlic cloves
- 2-inch piece ginger, peeled
- 2 tablespoons honey
- 1/4 cup rice wine vinegar
- 2 tablespoons extra-virgin olive oil

For the Stir-Fry
- 1/2 package extra-firm tofu
- 1 cup long-grain white rice
- 2 tablespoons extra-virgin olive oil
- 1 cup chopped broccoli
- 1 cup shredded carrots
- 3 scallions, finely chopped

Directions:

To Make the Sauce
1. Combine the garlic, ginger, honey, vinegar, and olive oil in a food processor, and purée until smooth.

To Make the Stir-Fry
1. Divide the tofu into small cubes, and press the excess moisture from the tofu using paper towels, repeating several times until dry.
2. In a medium pot, cook the rice according to package directions for about 20 minutes.
3. In a large skillet over medium heat, warm up the olive oil. Add the tofu to the pan in a single layer. Carefully add one quarter of the sauce to the pan and continue to cook, flipping the tofu only once or twice every 4 minutes, until it is well browned. With a slotted spoon, transfer the tofu to

a plate lined with paper towels to drain.

4. Add the broccoli to the pan. Cook, covered, stirring often, until fork-tender, about 5 minutes. Attach the carrots and continue to cook for an additional 3 minutes, until softened. Add the remaining sauce to the vegetables, return the tofu to the pan, and stir to mix. Garnish with scallions and serve over rice.

Nutrition Facts Per Serving:

Calories: 410 kcal
Total Fat: 18 g
Saturated Fat: 3 g
Cholesterol: 0 mg
Carbohydrates: 51 g
Fiber: 4 g
Protein: 13 g
Phosphorus: 222 mg
Potassium: 487 mg
Sodium: 51 mg

288. Vegetable Biryani

Preparation time: 10 minutes
Cooking time: 50 minutes
Servings: 4

Ingredients:

- 1 cup basmati rice
- 2 tablespoons olive oil or butter, divided
- 1/2 teaspoon curry powder
- 1/2 teaspoon cumin seeds
- 1/2 teaspoon coriander seeds
- 13/4 cups water plus 2/3 cup water, divided
- 1/2 sweet onion, chopped
- 2 garlic cloves, minced
- 1 teaspoon ground coriander
- 1/2 teaspoon ground cardamom
- 1/2 teaspoon ground cumin
- 1/4 teaspoon turmeric
- 1 cup cauliflower
- 1 cup green beans

- 1 carrot
- 1/4 cup chopped cilantro leaves

Directions:

1. In a small bowl, wash the rice until the water runs clear.
2. In a medium stockpot over medium heat, warm up 1 tablespoon of olive oil. Attach the curry powder, cumin seeds, and coriander seeds, stirring constantly, until fragrant, about 30 seconds. Attach the rice to the pot along with 1 3/4 cups of water. Set to a boil; reduce the heat, cover, and simmer for about 20 minutes.
3. In a skillet over medium heat, set the remaining tablespoon of olive oil. Add the onion, and cook for 6 to 8 minutes, until tender. Add the garlic and cook for an additional minute. Add the coriander, cardamom, cumin, and turmeric to the skillet, and stir constantly, toast until fragrant, about 1 minute. Add the cauliflower, beans, and carrots, stirring to coat, and cook for 2 to 3 minutes. Attach the remaining 2/3 cup of water to the pan, cover, and cook for 7 to 10 minutes, until the vegetables are just fork-tender.
4. Add the rice to the vegetables, and stir to blend. Serve topped with cilantro leaves.

Nutrition Facts Per Serving:

Calories: 470 kcal
Total Fat: 15.92 g
Saturated Fat: 1 g
Cholesterol: 4 mg
Carbohydrates: 74.39 g
Fiber: 3 g
Protein: 4 g
Phosphorus: 170 mg
Potassium: 500 mg
Sodium: 58.36 mg

289. Collard and Rice Stuffed Red Peppers

Preparation time: 10 minutes

Cooking time: 50 minutes

Servings: 4

Ingredients:

- 2 medium red bell peppers
- 2 tablespoons extra-virgin olive oil, divided
- Freshly ground black pepper
- 6 cups loosely packed collard greens, trimmed
- 1/2 sweet onion, chopped
- 3 garlic cloves, minced
- 1 cup cooked white rice or ½ cup basmati rice
- Juice of 1 lemon
- 1/4 cup toasted sunflower seeds, divided

Directions:

1. Preheat the oven to 400F.
2. Halve the peppers through the stems, and detach the seeds and stems. Garnish the inside and outside of the peppers with 1 tablespoon of olive oil and season with the pepper. Place the peppers cut-side down in a baking dish.
3. Bake them for 10 to 15 minutes, until just tender. Remove from the oven and flip the peppers cut-side up. Set aside, leaving the oven on.
4. In a large saucepan, Set 4 cups of water to a boil. Add the collard greens and cook until just tender, 5 to 7 minutes. Drain and rinse under cold water. Chop finely.
5. In a large skillet, heat the remaining tablespoon of olive oil over medium heat. Add the onion, and cook, stirring often, for 5 to 7 minutes, until it begins to brown. Add the garlic and cook until fragrant. Stir in the collard greens. Detach from the

heat, and stir in the cooked rice, half amount of sunflower seeds and lemon juice. Season with pepper.

6. Divide the filling between the pepper halves and top each pepper half with 1 tablespoon of the sunflower seeds.

7. Add 1/4 cup of water to the baking dish, cover with aluminum foil, and bake for 20 minutes, until heated through. Uncover and bake.

Nutrition Facts Per Serving:

Calories: 450 kcal
Total Fat: 9 g
Saturated Fat: 1 g
Cholesterol: 0 mg
Carbohydrates: 50 g
Fiber: 5 g
Protein: 8 g
Phosphorus: 147 mg
Potassium: 397 mg
Sodium: 20 mg

290. Stuffed Delicata Squash Boats with Bulgur and Vegetables

Preparation time: 10 minutes
Cooking time: 1 hour
Servings: 4

Ingredients:

- 2 small delicate squash, halved lengthwise and seeded
- 6 teaspoons extra-virgin olive oil, divided
- 1 cup bulgur
- 1/2 sweet onion, diced
- 2 tablespoons chili powder
- 1 cup canned black beans, drained and rinsed
- 1/2 cup frozen or fresh corn kernels
- 2 scallions, thinly sliced, for garnish

Directions:

1. Preheat the oven to 425F.

311

2. Brush the cut squash with 2 teaspoons of olive oil and place cut-side down on a baking sheet. Cook for 25 to 30 minutes, until the flesh is tender.

3. Meanwhile, in a saucepan, bring the bulgur and 2 cups of water to a boil. Lower the heat, covers, and simmers for 12 to 15 minutes, until the liquid is absorbed. Drain well.

4. In a large skillet, set the remaining 4 teaspoons of olive oil over medium heat. Cook the onion for 4 to 5 minutes, until it just starts to brown. Stir in the chili powder, black beans, and corn. Stir in the bulgur, and cook for an additional minute.

5. Divide the filling between the squash halves, sprinkle with scallions, and serve.

Nutrition Facts Per Serving:

Calories: 591.67 kcal
Total Fat: 17.1 g

Carbs: 103.16 g
Protein: 17.87 g
Sodium: 573.46 mg
Potassium: 700 mg
Phosphorus: 340 mg

291. Barley and Roasted Vegetable Bowl

Preparation time: 15 minutes

Cooking time: 1 hour

Servings: 4

Ingredients:

- 2 small Asian eggplants, diced
- 2 small zucchini, diced
- 1/2 red bell pepper, chopped
- 1/2 sweet onion, cut into wedges
- 2 tablespoons extra-virgin olive oil, divided
- Freshly ground black pepper
- 1 cup barley
- Juice of 1 lemon
- 3 garlic cloves, minced

312

- 1/4 cup basil leaves, roughly chopped
- 1/4 cup crumbled feta cheese
- 2 cups arugula or mixed baby salad greens

Directions:

1. Preheat the oven to 425F.
2. In a medium bowl, toss the eggplant, zucchini, bell pepper, and onion with 1 tablespoon of olive oil, and arrange the vegetables in a single layer on a baking sheet. Season with pepper.
3. Roast the vegetables for about 25 minutes, stirring once or twice, until they are browned and tender. Set aside.
4. Meanwhile, in a medium pot, add the barley and 2 cups of water. Bring to a boil, reduce the heat to simmer, cover, and cook for 20 minutes. Turn off the heat, and let rest for 10 minutes. Fluff with a fork, and drain any remaining water.
5. In a small bowl, whisk the lemon juice, garlic, and remaining tablespoon of olive oil.
6. Toss the vegetables with the barley, and then mix together with the lemon-garlic dressing. Right before serving, stir in the basil, feta cheese, and salad greens.

Nutrition Facts Per Serving:

Calories: 447.62 kcal
Total Fat: 19.84 g
Carbs: 60.55 g
Protein: 12.9g
Sodium: 244 mg
Potassium: 880 mg
phosphorus: 230 mg

Soups and Stews

292. French Onion Soup

Preparation time: 10 minutes

Cooking time: 30 minutes

Servings: 5

Ingredients:

- 2 tablespoons unsalted butter
- 4 Vidalia onions, sliced thin
- 2 cups Easy Chicken Stock
- 2 cups water
- 1 tablespoon chopped fresh thyme
- Freshly ground black pepper

Directions:

1. Dissolve the butter.
2. Attach the onions to the saucepan and cook them slowly, stirring frequently, for about 10 minutes.
3. Attach the chicken stock and water, and bring the soup to a boil.
4. Reduce the heat to low and simmer the soup for 15 minutes.
5. Stir in the thyme and season the soup with pepper.
6. Serve piping hot.

Nutrition Facts Per Serving:

Calories: 120 kcal
Fat: 6 g
Carbohydrates: 7 g
Phosphorus: 22 mg
Potassium: 192 mg
Sodium: 57 mg
Protein: 2 g

293. Cream of Watercress Soup

Preparation time: 15 minutes

Cooking time: 1 hour

Servings: 5

Ingredients:

- 6 garlic cloves
- 1/2 teaspoon olive oil
- 1 teaspoon unsalted butter

- 1/2 sweet onion, chopped
- 4 cups chopped watercress
- 1/4 cup chopped fresh parsley
- 3 cups water
- 1/4 cup lite cooking cream
- 1 tablespoon freshly squeezed lemon juice
- Freshly ground black pepper

Directions:

1. Preheat the oven to 400F.
2. Bring the garlic on a sheet of aluminum foil. Mizzle with olive oil and fold the foil into a little packet. Place the packet in a pie plate and roast the garlic for about 20 minutes or until very soft.
3. Remove the garlic from the oven; set aside to cool.
4. In a large saucepan over medium-high heat, melt the butter. Sauté the onion for about 4 minutes or until soft. Add the watercress and parsley; sauté 5 minutes.
5. Stir in the water and roasted garlic pulp. Set the soup to a boil, and then reduce the heat to low.
6. Stew the soup for about 20 minutes or until the vegetables are soft.
7. Cool the soup for about 5 minutes, then purée in batches in a food processor along with the heavy cream.
8. Transfer the soup to the pot, and set over low heat until warmed through.
9. Add the lemon juice and season with pepper.

Nutrition Facts Per Serving:

Calories: 150 kcal
Fat: 8 g
Carbohydrates: 5 g
Sodium: 23 mg
Phosphorus: 46 mg
Potassium: 380 mg
Protein: 2 g

294. Curried Cauliflower Soup

Preparation time: 10 minutes

Cooking time: 40 minutes

Servings: 6

Ingredients:

- 1 teaspoon unsalted butter
- 1 small, sweet onion, chopped
- 2 teaspoons minced garlic
- 1 small head cauliflower
- 3 cups water
- 2 teaspoons curry powder
- 1/2 cup light sour cream
- 3 tablespoons chopped fresh cilantro

Directions:

1. In a large saucepan, warm up the butter over medium-high heat and sauté the onion and garlic for about 3 minutes or until softened.
2. Add the cauliflower, water, and curry powder.
3. Set the soup to a boil, and then reduce the heat to low and simmer.
4. Pour the soup into a food processor and purée until the soup is smooth and creamy (or use a large bowl and a handheld immersion blender).
5. Transfer the soup back into a saucepan and stir in the sour cream and cilantro.
6. Heat the soup on medium-low for about 5 minutes or until warmed through.

Nutrition Facts Per Serving:

Calories 196.2 kcal

Total Fat: 9.1g

Carbs: 24.77 g

Protein: 8.43 g

Sodium: 164.49 mg

Potassium: 900 mg

Phosphorus: 130 mg

295. Roasted Red Pepper and Eggplant Soup

Preparation time: 20 minutes

Cooking time: 40 minutes

Servings: 6

Ingredients:

- 1 small, sweet onion, cut into quarters
- 2 small red bell peppers, halved
- 2 cups cubed eggplant
- 2 garlic cloves, crushed
- 1 tablespoon olive oil
- 1 cup Easy Chicken Stock (here)
- Water
- 1/4 cup chopped fresh basil
- Freshly ground black pepper

Directions:

1. Preheat the oven to 350F.
2. Put the onions, red peppers, eggplant, and garlic in a large ovenproof baking dish.
3. Drizzle the vegetables with the olive oil.
4. Roast the vegetables.
5. Cool the vegetables slightly and remove the skin from the peppers.
6. Purée the vegetables in batches in a food processor (or in a large bowl, using a handheld immersion blender) with the chicken stock.
7. Transfer the soup to a medium pot and add enough water to reach the desired thickness. Heat the soup to a simmer and add the basil.
8. Season with pepper and serve.

Nutrition Facts Per Serving:

Calories: 280kcal

Fat: 2 g

Total Fat: 9.14 g

Carbs: 21.45 g

Sodium: 183.45 mg

Potassium: 600 mg

296. Traditional Chicken-vegetable Soup

Preparation time: 20 minutes

Cooking time: 35 minutes

Servings: 6

Ingredients:

- 1 tablespoon unsalted butter
- 1/2 sweet onion, diced
- 2 teaspoons minced garlic
- 2 celery stalks, chopped
- 1 carrot, diced
- 1 cup chopped cooked chicken breast
- 1 cup Easy Chicken Stock (here)
- 4 cups water
- 1 teaspoon chopped fresh thyme
- Freshly ground black pepper
- 2 tablespoons chopped fresh parsley

Directions:

1. Dissolve the butter.
2. Simmer the onion and garlic until softened.
3. Put the celery, carrot, chicken, chicken stock, and water.
4. Set the soup to a boil until the vegetables are tender.
5. Attach the thyme; simmer the soup for 2 minutes.
6. Flavor with pepper and serve topped with parsley.

Nutrition Facts Per Serving:

Calories: 246.18 kcal

Fat: 13.67g

Carbohydrates: 2 g

Protein: 18.63 g

Sodium: 298.51 mg

Potassium: 550 mg

Phosphorus: 180 mg

297. Turkey and Lemon-grass Soup

Preparation Time: 5 minutes

Cooking Time: 40 minutes

Servings: 4

Ingredients:

- 1 fresh lime
- 1/4 cup fresh basil leaves
- 1 tbsp. cilantro
- 1 cup chestnuts
- 1 tbsp. coconut oil
- 1 thumb-size minced ginger piece
- 2 chopped scallions
- 1 finely chopped green chili
- 4oz. skinless and sliced turkey breasts
- 1 minced garlic clove, minced
- 1/2 finely sliced stick lemon-grass
- 1 chopped white onion, chopped
- 4 cups water

Directions:

1. Crush the lemon-grass, cilantro, chili, 1 tbsp. oil, and basil leaves in a blender or pestle and mortar to form a paste.
2. Heat a large pan/wok with 1 tbsp. olive oil on high heat.
3. Sauté the onions, garlic, and ginger until soft.
4. Add the turkey and brown each side for 4-5 minutes.
5. Add the broth and stir.
6. Now add the paste and stir.
7. Next, add the chestnuts, turn down the heat slightly, and simmer for 25-30 minutes or until the turkey is thoroughly cooked through.
8. Serve hot with the green onion sprinkled over the top.

Nutrition Facts Per Serving:

Calories 340.83kcal

Total Fat 12.76g

Carbs 42.11g

Protein: 15.63 g

Sodium: 49.97 mg

Potassium: 720 mg

Phosphorus: 210 mg

298. Herbed Soup with Black Beans

Preparation Time: 10 minutes

Cooking Time: 10 minutes

Servings: 4

Ingredients:

- 2 tbsp. tomato paste
- 1/3 cup Poland pepper, charred, peeled, seeded and chopped
- 2 cups vegetable stock
- 1/4 tsp. cumin
- 1/2 tsp. paprika
- 1/2 tsp. dried oregano
- 2 tsp. fresh garlic, minced
- 1 cup onion, small diced
- 1 tbsp. extra-virgin olive oil
- 1.5 oz can black beans

Directions:

1. On medium fire, place a soup pot and heat oil. Attach onion and sauté until translucent and soft, around 4-5 minutes. Add garlic, cook for 2 minutes.
2. Attach the rest of the ingredients and bring to a simmer. Once simmering, turn off the fire and transfer to a blender. Puree ingredients until smooth.

Nutrition Facts Per Serving:

Calories: 148.73 kcal

Total Fat: 7.69 g

Carbs: 18.13 g

Sugars: 7.08 g

Protein: 3.73 g

Sodium: 816.43 mg

Potassium: 440 mg

Phosphorus: 37 mg

299. Tofu Soup

Preparation Time: 5 minutes
Cooking Time: 10 minutes
Servings: 2

Ingredients:

- 1 tbsp. miso paste
- 1/8 cup cubed soft tofu
- 1 chopped green onion
- 1/4 cup sliced Shiitake mushrooms
- 3 cups Renali stock
- 1 tbsp. soy sauce

Directions:

1. Take a saucepan, pour the stock into this pan and let it boil on high heat. Reduce heat to medium and let this stock simmer. Add mushrooms to this stock and cook for almost 3 minutes.
2. Take a bowl and mix soy sauce (reduced salt) and miso paste together in this bowl. Add this mixture and tofu to stock. Simmer for nearly 5 minutes and serve with chopped green onion.

Nutrition Facts Per Serving:

Calories: 129 kcal

Fat 7.8 g

Sodium 484 mg

Potassium 435 mg

Protein: 11 g

Carbs: 5.5 g

Phosphorus: 73.2 mg

300. Turkey-bulgur Soup

Preparation time: 25 minutes
Cooking time: 45 minutes
Servings: 6

Ingredients:

- 1 teaspoon olive oil
- 2 oz. cooked ground turkey, 93% lean
- 1/2 sweet onion, chopped
- 1 teaspoon minced garlic
- 4 cups water
- 1 cup Easy Chicken Stock (here)
- 1 celery stalk, chopped

- 1 carrot, sliced thin
- 1/2 cup shredded green cabbage
- 1/2 cup bulgur
- 2 dried bay leaves
- 2 tablespoons chopped fresh parsley
- 1 teaspoon chopped fresh sage
- 1 teaspoon chopped fresh thyme
- Pinch red pepper flakes
- Freshly ground black pepper

Directions:

1. Heat the olive oil. Sauté the turkey until the meat is cooked through.
2. Attach the onion and garlic and sauté for about 3 minutes or until the vegetables are softened. Attach the water, chicken stock, celery, carrot, cabbage, bulgur, and bay leaves.
3. Set the soup to a boil and then reduce the heat to low and simmer until the bulgur and vegetables are tender.
4. Detach the bay leaves and stir in the parsley, sage, thyme, and red pepper flakes.
5. Season with pepper and serve.

Nutrition Facts Per Serving:

Calories: 277.93 kcal
Total Fat: 9.57 g
Carbs: 38.59 g
Protein: 11.91 g
Sodium: 259.82 mg
Potassium: 550 mg
Phosphorus: 160 mg

301. Mediterranean Vegetable Soup

Preparation Time: 5 minutes
Cooking Time: 30 minutes
Servings: 4

Ingredients:

- 1 tbsp. oregano
- 2 minced garlic cloves
- 1 tsp. black pepper

- 1 diced zucchini
- 1 cup diced eggplant
- 4 cups water
- 1 diced red pepper
- 1 tbsp. extra-virgin olive oil
- 1 diced red onion

Directions:

1. Soak the vegetables in warm water before use.
2. In a large pot, add the oil, chopped onion, and minced garlic.
3. Sweat for 5 minutes on low heat.
4. Add the other vegetables to the onions and cook for 7-8 minutes.
5. Add the stock to the pan and bring to a boil on high heat.
6. Stir in the herbs, reduce the heat, and simmer for a further 20 minutes or until thoroughly cooked through.
7. Season with pepper to serve.

Nutrition Facts Per Serving:

Calories: 152 kcal

Protein: 1 g

Carbs: 6 g

Fat: 3 g

Sodium 3 mg

Potassium 229 mg

Phosphorus: 45 mg

302. Onion Soup

Preparation Time: 15 minutes
Cooking Time: 45 minutes
Servings: 6

Ingredients:

- 2 tbsp. chicken stock
- 1 cup chopped shiitake mushrooms
- 1 tbsp. minced chives
- 3 tsps. beef bouillon
- 1 tsp. grated ginger root
- 1/2 chopped carrot
- 1 cup sliced Portobello mushrooms
- 1 chopped onion
- 1/2 chopped celery stalk
- 2 quarts' water

- 1/4 tsp. minced garlic

Directions:

1. Take a saucepan and combine carrot, onion, celery, garlic, mushrooms (some mushrooms), and ginger in this pan. Add water, beef bouillon, and chicken stock to this pan. Put this pot on high heat and let it boil. Decrease flame to medium and cover this pan to cook for almost 45 minutes.

2. Put all remaining mushrooms in one separate pot. Once the boiling mixture is completely done, put one strainer over this new bowl with mushrooms and strain cooked soup in this pot over mushrooms. Discard solid-strained materials.

3. Serve delicious broth with yummy mushrooms in small bowls and sprinkle chives over each bowl.

Nutrition Facts Per Serving:

Calories: 90.58 kcal
Total Fat: 1.09 g
Carbs: 17.44 g
Protein: 6.27 g
Sodium: 77.54 mg
Potassium: 710 mg
Phosphorus: 210 mg

303. Roasted Red Pepper Soup

Preparation Time: 30 minutes

Cooking Time: 35 minutes

Servings: 4

Ingredients:

- 4 cups low-sodium chicken broth
- 3 red peppers
- 2 medium onions
- 3 tbsp. lemon juice
- 1 tbsp. finely minced lemon zest
- A pinch of cayenne pepper
- 1/4 tsp. cinnamon

- 1/2 cup finely minced fresh cilantro

Directions:

1. In a medium stockpot, consolidate each one of the fixings except for the cilantro and warmth to the point of boiling over excessive warm temperature. Diminish the warmth and stew, ordinarily secured, for around 30 minutes, till thickened. Cool marginally. Utilizing a hand blender or nourishment processor, puree the soup. Include the cilantro and tenderly heat.

Nutrition Facts Per Serving:

Calories: 175.67 kcal
Total Fat: 3.62 g
Carbs: 29.32 g
Sugars: 13.54 g
Protein: 12.81 g
Sodium: 157.85 mg
Potassium: 1000 mg

Phosphorus: 200 mg

304. Ground Beef and Rice Soup

Preparation time: 15 minutes
Cooking time: 1 ¼ hours
Servings: 6

Ingredients:

- 2 oz. extra-lean ground beef
- 1/2 small, sweet onion, chopped
- 1 teaspoon minced garlic
- 2 cups water
- 1 cup homemade low-sodium beef broth
- 1/2 cup long-grain white rice, uncooked
- 1 celery stalk, chopped
- 1/2 cup fresh green beans
- 1 teaspoon chopped fresh thyme
- Freshly ground black pepper

Directions:

1. Cook beef. Sauté, stirring often, for about 6 minutes until the beef is completely browned.
2. Drain off the excess fat and add the onion and garlic to the saucepan.
3. Sauté the vegetables until they are softened for 5 minutes.
4. Add the water, beef broth, and celery and simmer for 40 minutes.
5. Add rice for another 20 minutes
6. Add the green beans and thyme and simmer for 3 minutes.
7. Remove the soup from the heat and season with pepper.

Nutrition Facts Per Serving:

Calories: 235.55 kcal
Total Fat: 1.93 g
Carbs: 42.09 g
Protein: 11.48 g
Sodium: 244.87 mg
Potassium: 340 mg
Phosphorus: 141 mg

305. Red Pepper and Brie Soup

Preparation Time: 10 minutes

Cooking Time: 35 minutes

Servings: 4

Ingredients:

- 1 tsp. paprika
- 1 tsp. cumin
- 1 chopped red onion
- 2 chopped garlic cloves
- 1/4 cup crumbled brie
- 2 tbsps. extra virgin olive oil
- 4 chopped red bell peppers
- 4 cups water

Directions:

1. Warmth the oil in a pot over medium heat.
2. Sweat the onions and peppers for 5 minutes.
3. Add the garlic cloves, cumin, and paprika and sauté for 3-4 minutes.
4. Add the water and allow to boil before turning the

heat down to simmer for 30 minutes.

5. Detach from the heat and allow to cool slightly.
6. Put the mixture in a food processor and blend until smooth.
7. Pour into serving bowls and add the crumbled brie to the top with a little black pepper.
8. Enjoy!

Nutrition Facts Per Serving:

Calories: 152 kcal
Protein: 3 g
Carbs: 8 g
Fat: 11 g
Sodium: 66 mg
Potassium: 270 mg
Phosphorus: 207 mg

306. Herbed Cabbage Stew

Preparation time: 20 minutes
Cooking time: 35 minutes
Servings: 6

Ingredients:

- 1 teaspoon unsalted butter
- 1/2 large, sweet onion, chopped
- 1 teaspoon minced garlic
- 6 cups shredded green cabbage
- 3 celery stalks, chopped with the leafy tops
- 1 scallion, chopped
- 2 tablespoons chopped fresh parsley
- 2 tablespoons freshly squeezed lemon juice
- 1 tablespoon chopped fresh thyme
- 1 teaspoon chopped savory
- 1 teaspoon chopped fresh oregano
- Water

- 1 cup fresh green beans
- Freshly ground black pepper

Directions:

1. In a medium stockpot over medium-high heat, dissolve the butter.
2. Sauté the onion and garlic in the melted butter for about 3 minutes or until the vegetables are softened.
3. Add the cabbage, celery, scallion, parsley, lemon juice, thyme, savory, and oregano to the pot, and pour enough water to cover the vegetables by about 4 inches.
4. Set the soup to a boil, reduce the heat to low, and simmer the soup for 10 minutes until the vegetables are tender.
5. Add the green beans and simmer for 3 minutes.
6. Season with pepper.

Nutrition Facts Per Serving:

Calories: 107.65 kcal
Total Fat: 2.42 g
Carbs: 21.19 g
Sugars: 10.47 g
Protein: 4.21 g
Sodium: 104.94 mg
Potassium: 680 mg
Phosphorus: 90 mg

307. Paprika Pork Soup

Preparation Time: 5 minutes
Cooking Time: 35 minutes
Servings: 2

Ingredients:

- 4 oz. sliced pork loin
- 1 tsp. black pepper
- 2 minced garlic cloves
- 3 cups water
- 1 tbsp. extra-virgin olive oil
- 1 chopped onion
- 1 tbsp. paprika

Directions:

1. In a large pot, attach the oil, chopped onion, and minced garlic.
2. Sauté for 5 minutes on low heat.
3. Add the pork slices to the onions and cook for 7-8 minutes or until browned.
4. Add the water to the pan and bring to a boil on high heat.
5. Season with pepper to serve.

Nutrition Facts Per Serving:

Calories: 250 kcal
Protein: 13 g
Carbs: 10 g
Fat: 9 g
Sodium: 269 mg
Potassium: 486 mg
Phosphorus: 158 mg

308. Winter Chicken Stew

Preparation time: 20 minutes
Cooking time: 50 minutes
Servings: 6

Ingredients:

- 1 tablespoon olive oil
- 1-pound boneless chicken
- 1/2 sweet onion, chopped
- 1 tablespoon minced garlic
- 2 cups Easy Chicken Stock (here)
- 1 cup plus 2 tablespoons water
- 1 carrot, sliced
- 2 celery stalks, sliced
- 1 turnip, sliced thin
- 1 tablespoon chopped fresh thyme
- 1 teaspoon finely chopped fresh rosemary
- 2 teaspoons cornstarch
- Freshly ground black pepper

Directions:

1. Heat the olive oil.
2. Sauté the chicken for about 6 minutes or until it is lightly browned, stirring often.
3. Attach the onion and garlic and sauté for 3 minutes.
4. Add the chicken stock, 1 cup water, carrot, celery, and turnip and bring the stew to a boil.
5. Set the heat to low and simmer or until the chicken is cooked through and tender for about 30 minutes.
6. Add the thyme and rosemary and simmer for 3 more minutes.
7. In a small bowl, toss together the 2 tablespoons of water and the cornstarch, and add the mixture to the stew.
8. Stir to incorporate the cornstarch mixture and cook for 3 to 4 minutes or until the stew thickens.
9. Detach from the heat and season with pepper.

Nutrition Facts Per Serving:

Calories: 482.34 kcal
Total Fat: 16.21 g
Carbs: 22.35 g
Protein 58.49g
Sodium: 566.84 mg
Potassium: 1371.32 mg
Phosphorus: 560 mg

309. Creamy Pumpkin Soup

> **Preparation Time: 10 minutes**
> **Cooking Time: 20 minutes**
> **Servings: 4**

Ingredients:

- 1 onion, chopped
- 1 slice of bacon
- 2 tsp. ground ginger
- 1 tsp. cinnamon
- 1 cup applesauce
- 3 1/2 cups low sodium chicken broth
- 1.5 oz canned pumpkin

- Pepper to taste
- 1/2 cup light sour cream

Directions:

1. On medium-high fire, place a soup pot and add bacon once hot. Sauté until crispy, around 4 minutes. Discard bacon fat before continuing to cook. Add ginger, applesauce, chicken broth, and pumpkin. Lightly season with pepper. Set to a simmer and cook for 11 minutes. Taste and adjust seasoning. Turn off fire, stir in sour cream and mix well.

Nutrition Facts Per Serving:

Calories: 320.91
Fat: 14.01 g
Fiber: 10 g
Carbs: 36 g
Protein: 10 g
Sodium: 262.9 mg
Potassium: 700 mg
Phosphorus: 200 mg

310. Roasted Beef Stew

Preparation time: 30 minutes
Cooking time: 1 ½ hour
Servings: 6

Ingredients:

- 1/4 cup all-purpose flour
- 1 teaspoon freshly ground black pepper
- Pinch cayenne pepper
- 1/2-pound boneless beef
- 2 tablespoons olive oil
- 1/2 sweet onion, chopped
- 2 teaspoons minced garlic
- 1 cup homemade beef stock
- 1 cup plus 2 tablespoons water
- 1 carrot, cut into 1/2-inch chunks
- 2 celery stalks, chopped with greens
- 1 teaspoon chopped fresh thyme
- 1 teaspoon cornstarch
- 2 tablespoons chopped fresh parsley

Directions:

1. Preheat the oven to 350F.
2. Set the flour, black pepper, and cayenne pepper in a large plastic freezer bag and toss to merge.
3. Attach the beef chunks to the bag and toss to season.
4. Heat the olive oil.
5. Sauté the beef chunks until they are lightly browned for about 10 minutes.
6. Detach the beef from the pot and set aside on a plate.
7. Attach the onion and garlic to the pot and sauté.
8. Attach 1 cup water, the beef drippings on the plate, the carrot, celery, and thyme.
9. Seal the pot tightly with a lid or aluminum foil and place in the oven.
10. Bake the stew until the meat is very tender for about 1 hour.
11. Flavor the stew with black pepper and serve topped with parsley.

Nutrition Facts Per Serving:

Calories: 392.73 kcal
Total Fat: 21.55 g
Carbs: 22.47 g
Protein: 28.31 g
Sodium: 407.68 mg
Potassium: 900 mg
Phosphorus: 310 mg

311. Spring Vegetable Soup

Preparation Time: 10 minutes
Cooking Time: 1 hour
Servings: 4

Ingredients:

- Vegetable broth (low-sodium): 4 cups
- Fresh green beans: 1 cup
- Half cup carrots
- Celery: 3/4 cup
- Garlic powder: 1 teaspoon
- Half cup onion

- Half cup mushrooms
- Olive oil: 2 tablespoons
- Dried oregano leaves: 1 teaspoon
- 1/4 teaspoon salt
- Half cup frozen corn

Directions:

1. Trim the green beans and chop into two-inch pieces
2. Chop up the vegetables.
3. In a pot, heat olive oil, sauté the onion and celery till tender.
4. Then add the remaining ingredients with the broth.
5. Let it boil and cook for about 40 minutes.
6. Lower the heat and let it simmer. Then serve.

Nutrition Facts Per Serving:

Calories: 144 kcal
Protein: 2 g
Carbohydrates: 13 g
Fat: 6 g
Sodium: 262 mg
Potassium: 365 mg

Phosphorus: 108 mg
Calcium: 48 mg
Fiber: 3.4 g

312. Leek and Carrot Soup

Preparation Time: 15 minutes
Cooking Time: 25 minutes
Servings: 4

Ingredients:

- leek
- 3/4 cup diced and boiled carrots
- 1 garlic clove
- 1 tbsp olive oil
- Crushed pepper to taste
- cups low sodium chicken stock
- Chopped parsley for garnish
- 1 bay leaf
- 1/4 tsp. ground cumin

Directions:

1. Trim off and take away a portion of the coarse inexperienced portions of the leek. At that factor,

reduce daintily and flush altogether in water. Channel properly. Warmth the oil in an extensively based pot. Include the leek and garlic, and sear over low warmth for two-3 minutes, till sensitive. Include the inventory, inlet leaf, cumin, and pepper.

2. Warmth the mixture to the point of boiling, mixing constantly. Include carrots and stew for 13 minutes. Modify the flavoring, eliminate the inlet leaf, and serve sprinkled with slashed parsley. To make a pureed soup, manner the soup in a blender or nourishment processor till smooth. Come again to the pan. Include 1/2 field milk. Bring to bubble and stew for 4 minutes.

Calories 119.6kcal

Total Fat 7.48g

Carbs 12.41g

Sugars 4.47g

Protein 1.88g

Sodium 112.65mg

potassium 250mg

phosphorus 37mg

313. Spaghetti Squash and Yellow Bell-Pepper Soup

Preparation Time: 10 minutes

Cooking Time: 45 minutes

Servings: 4

Ingredients:

- 2 diced yellow bell peppers
- 2 chopped large garlic cloves
- 1 peeled and cubed spaghetti squash
- 1 quartered and sliced onion

- 1 tbsp. dried thyme
- 1 tbsp. coconut oil
- 1 tsp. curry powder
- 4 cups water

Directions:

1. Warmth the oil over medium-high heat before sweating the onions and garlic for 3-4 minutes.
2. Sprinkle over the curry powder.
3. Attach the stock and bring to a boil over a high heat before adding the squash, pepper, and thyme.
4. Turn down the heat, cover, and allow to simmer for 25-30 minutes.
5. Continue to simmer until squash is soft if needed.
6. Allow cooling before blitzing in a blender/food processor until smooth.
7. Serve!

Nutrition Facts Per Serving:

Calories: 150 kcal

Protein: 2 g
Carbs: 17 g
Fat: 4 g
Sodium: 32 mg
Potassium: 365 mg
Phosphorus: 50 mg

314. Steakhouse Soup

Preparation Time: 15 minutes
Cooking Time: 25 minutes
Servings: 4

Ingredients:

- 2 tbsps. soy sauce
- 2 boneless and cubed chicken breast halves
- 1/4 lb. halved and trimmed snow peas
- 1 tbsp. minced ginger root
- 1 minced garlic clove
- 1 cup water
- 2 chopped green onions
- 3 cups chicken stock
- 1 chopped carrot
- 3 sliced mushrooms

Directions:

1. Take a pot and combine ginger, water, chicken stock, Soy sauce (reduced salt), and garlic in this pot. Let them boil on medium heat, mix in chicken pieces, and let them simmer on low heat for almost 15 minutes to tender chicken.

2. Stir in carrot and snow peas and simmer for almost 5 minutes. Add mushrooms to this blend and continue cooking to tender vegetables for nearly 3 minutes. Mix in the chopped onion and serve hot.

Nutrition Facts Per Serving:

Calories: 319 kcal
Carbs: 14 g
Fat: 15 g
Potassium: 225 mg
Protein: 29 g
Sodium: 389 mg
Phosphorous: 190 mg

315. Cauliflower Soup

Preparation Time: 5 minutes

Cooking Time: 30 minutes

Servings: 6

Ingredients:

- 1 teaspoon unsalted butter
- 1 small, chopped, sweet onion–
- 2 teaspoons minced garlic
- 1 small head cauliflower, cut into small florets
- 2 teaspoons curry powder
- Water to cover the cauliflower
- 1/2 cup light sour cream
- 3 tablespoons chopped fresh cilantro

Directions:

1. In a large saucepan, warm up the butter over medium-high heat and sauté the onion-garlic for about 3 minutes or until softened.

2. Add the cauliflower, water, and curry powder.
3. Set the soup to a boil, then reduce the heat to low and simmer for 20 minutes or until the cauliflower is tender.
4. Puree the soup until creamy and smooth with a hand mixer.
5. Transfer the soup back into a saucepan and stir in the sour cream and cilantro.
6. Warm the soup on medium heat for 5 minutes or until warmed through.

Nutrition Facts Per Serving:

Calories: 195.85 kcal
Total Fat: 9.09 g
Carbs: 24.71 g
Protein: 8.4 g
Sodium: 156.9 mg
Potassium: 1009 mg
Phosphorus: 190 mg

316. Kidney Diet Friendly Chicken Noodle Soup

Preparation Time: 10 minutes

Cooking Time: 25 minutes

Servings: 4

Ingredients:

- 1 cup cooked Chicken Breast
- Unsalted Butter: 1 tbsp.
- 1/2 cup of Chopped Celery
- Chicken Stock: 5 cups
- 1/2 tsp. Ground Basil
- 1/2 cup of chopped Onions
- Ground Black Pepper 1/4 tsp.
- Egg Noodles: 1 cup, Dry
- Sliced Carrots: 1 cup
- 1/2 tsp. Ground Oregano

Directions:

1. Chop up all the vegetables.

2. In a Dutch oven (5 quarts), melt butter over low heat.
3. Cook celery and onion for five minutes. Add in the carrots, oregano, chicken stock, basil, pepper, chicken and noodles.
4. Let it boil for 10 minutes.
5. Serve hot.

Nutrition Facts Per Serving:

Calories: 479.41 kcal
Total Fat: 17.49 g
Carbs: 51.84 g
Protein: 27.74 g
Sodium: 953.01 mg
Potassium: 1100 mg
Phosphorus: 370 mg

317. Renal-friendly Cream of Mushroom Soup

Preparation Time: 5 minutes
Cooking Time: 15 minutes
Servings: 2

Ingredients:

- Minced mushrooms: 1/4 cup
- Unsalted butter: 3 tbsp.
- All-purpose flour: 2 and a half tbsp.
- Sea salt, pepper to taste
- Low sodium chicken broth: half cup
- Finely chopped onion: 1/4 cup
- Unsweetened almond milk: half cup

Directions:

1. In a skillet, dissolve the butter and sauté onions till tender
2. Add mushrooms and cook for five minutes.

Add flour and cook for 1 minute and stir for frying

3. Add in milk and broth mix continuously.
4. Let it simmer until it becomes thick for five minutes.

Nutrition Facts Per Serving:

Calories: 191 kcal
Total Fat: 18.2 g
Cholesterol: 45.8 mg
Sodium: 162.8 mg
Carbohydrates: 10.2 g
Dietary Fiber: 0.9 g
Protein: 2.1 g
Iron: 1 mg
Potassium: 123.7 mg

318. Rotisserie Chicken Noodle Soup

Preparation Time: 10 minutes
Cooking Time: 15 minutes
Servings: 2

Ingredients:

- Carrots: 1 cup, sliced
- 2 cups cooked rotisserie chicken
- 1/2 cup of onion, chopped
- Celery: 1 cup, sliced
- Chicken broth (low-sodium): 4 cups
- Fresh parsley: 3 tablespoons
- Wide noodles: 6 ounces, uncooked

Directions:

1. Set the bones out of the chicken and cut them into one-inch pieces. Take 2 cups of chicken pieces.

2. In a large pot, add chicken broth and let it boil for 10 minutes.
3. Add noodles and vegetables to the broth.
4. Let it boil and cook for 15 minutes. Make sure noodles are tender.
5. Serve with chopped parsley on top.

Nutrition Facts Per Serving:

Calories: 569.02 kcal
Total Fat: 13.38 g
Carbs: 73.68 g
Protein: 36.8 g
Sodium: 1654.6 mg
Potassium: 1000 mg
Phosphorus: 320 mg

319. Quick and Easy Ground Beef Soup

Preparation Time: 10 minutes
Cooking Time: 1 hour
Servings: 2

Ingredients:

- Frozen mixed vegetables: 3 cups
- 1/2 cup of onion, chopped
- Beef broth (reduced-sodium): 1 cup
- White rice: 1/3 cup, uncooked
- Lemon pepper (no salt): 2 teaspoons, seasoning
- 2 cups lean ground beef
- Light or 40% fat only sour cream: 1 tablespoon
- Water: 2 cups

Directions:

1. In a pot, sauté onion, brown the beef. Drain the fat.
2. Add all the remaining ingredients and seasoning.

3. Add water and Let it boil to cook beef first for 30 minutes.
4. Lower the heat, add water, cover it and cook for 20 minutes.
5. Turn off the heat, add sour cream.

Nutrition Facts Per Serving:

Calories: 430 kcal
Protein: 20 g
Carbohydrates: 19 g
Fat: 8 g
Cholesterol: 52 mg
Sodium: 170 mg
Potassium: 448 mg
Phosphorus: 210 mg
Calcium: 43 mg
Fiber: 4.3 g

320. Chicken and Dill Soup

Preparation Time: 10 minutes

Cooking Time: 1 ¼ hour

Servings: 6

Ingredients:

- ½ Pound whole chicken.
- Carrots, 1 pound, sliced
- Low-sodium veggie stock for 6 cups
- 1 cup of yellow, diced onion
- A pinch of black pepper and Salt
- 2 dill teaspoons, diced
- 1/2 cup red, minced onion

Directions:

1. Set the chicken in a saucepan; add the water to coat it. Let it simmer for 1 hour.
2. Take the chicken out, remove the bones, strip the meat, strain the soup, put everything back in the saucepan, hot it over a

moderate flame, and add the chicken.

3. Add the carrots, red onion, a pinch of Salt, yellow onion, black pepper, and dill, roast for fifteen minutes, and put in bowls.

Nutrition Facts Per Serving:

Calories: 360 kcal
Protein: 21 g
Carbohydrates: 28 g
Fat: 11 g
Cholesterol: 45 mg
Sodium: 900 mg
Potassium: 1200 mg
Phosphorus: 252 mg
Calcium: 183 mg
Fiber: 3.3g

321. Maryland's Eastern Shore Cream of Crab Soup

Preparation Time: 10 minutes

Cooking Time: 10 minutes

Servings: 4

Ingredients:

- 0.25 cup non-dairy creamer
- Unsalted butter: 1 tablespoon
- Old bay seasoning: 1/4 teaspoon
- 2 cups crab meat
- Chicken broth (low-sodium): 4 cups
- 1 medium onion
- Cornstarch: 2 tablespoons
- Black pepper: 1/8 teaspoon
- Dill weed: 1/8 teaspoon

Directions:

1. In a large pot, dissolve butter over medium flame.

2. Add chopped onion to the pot. Cook until tender.
3. Add crab meat—Cook for 2 to 3 minutes, stir often.
4. Add chicken broth, let it boil, turn heat down to low.
5. Mix starch and creamer in a bowl, mix well.
6. Add the mixture to the soup, increase the heat, stir until the soup thickens and gets to a boil.
7. Add Old Bay, dill weed, pepper to soup.

Nutrition Facts Per Serving:

Calories: 390 kcal
Protein: 31 g
Carbohydrates: 7 g
Fat: 6 g
Cholesterol: 53 mg
Sodium: 212 mg
Potassium: 700 mg
Phosphorus: 400 mg
Calcium: 86 mg
Fiber: 0.4 g

322. Old Fashioned Salmon Soup

Preparation Time: 10 minutes

Cooking Time: 30 minutes

Servings: 4

Ingredients:

- Chicken broth, reduced-sodium: 2 cups
- Unsalted butter: 2 tablespoons
- 1/2 cup onion, chopped
- Sockeye salmon: 4 oz., cooked
- One medium carrot, chopped
- 1% low-fat milk: 2 cups
- 1/2 cup celery, chopped
- Black pepper: 1/8 teaspoon
- Water: 1/4 cup
- Cornstarch: 1/4 cup

Directions:

1. In a large pot, dissolve the butter and cook the vegetables on low, medium flame until tender.
2. Add the cooked salmon chunks. Add in the milk, broth, pepper.
3. Let it simmer on low heat.
4. Mix water and cornstarch. Keep stirring and slowly add the cornstarch mix.
5. Cook until the soup becomes thick.
6. Simmer for 5 minutes and serve.

Nutrition Facts Per Serving:

Calories: 380.8 kcal

Total Fat: 16.28 g

Carbs: 33.99 g

Protein: 25.15 g

Sodium: 754.07 mg

Potassium: 1000 mg

Phosphorus: 330 mg

323. The Kale and Green Lettuce Soup

Preparation Time: 5 minutes

Cooking Time: 10 minutes

Servings: 4

Ingredients:

- 2 tbsp. coconut oil
- 8 oz. kale, chopped
- 2 1/3 cups coconut almond milk
- 1 cup water.
- Sunflower seeds and pepper to taste

Directions:

1. Place a skillet and set it over medium heat.
2. Attach kale and sauté for 2-3 minutes
3. Add kale to the blender.
4. Add water, spices, coconut almond milk to the blender as well.
5. Blend until smooth and pour the mix into a bowl.
6. Serve and enjoy!

Nutrition Facts Per Serving:

Calories: 293 kcal

Fat: 24 g

Carbohydrates: 7 g

Protein: 4.2 g

Phosphorus: 110 mg

Potassium: 500 mg

Sodium: 105 mg

324. Turkey, Wild Rice, and Mushroom Soup

Preparation time: 15 minutes

Cooking time: 35 minutes

Servings: 6

Ingredients:

- Turkey: 1 cup, cooked, shredded
- 1/2 cup of onion, chopped
- 1/2 cup of carrots, chopped
- 2 garlic cloves, minced
- Chicken broth, low-sodium: 3 cups

- 1/2 cup of red bell pepper, chopped
- 1/2 cup of uncooked wild rice,
- Olive oil: 1 tablespoon
- 1/2 teaspoon salt
- 2 bay leaves
- Herb seasoning: 1/4 teaspoon
- Dried thyme: 1-and half teaspoon
- Black pepper: 1/4 teaspoon
- 1/2 cup of sliced mushrooms

Directions:

1. In a pot, boil the one and 3/4 broth over medium flame.
2. Add rice to the broth and cook. Let it boil. Turn the heat down. Close and let it simmer until all broth is absorbed for about 20 minutes.
3. In a Dutch oven, heat oil, add garlic, bell pepper, onion, and carrots. Sauté them.
4. Add the mushroom to the vegetables, and then add the broth, turkey, herb seasoning, salt, pepper, thyme, and bay leaves. Cook until it is well heated. Stir often.
5. Before adding the rice, take out the bay leaves. Cook for a minute and serve.

Nutrition Facts Per Serving:

Calories: 370 kcal
Protein: 23 g
Carbohydrate: 15 g
Fat: 5 g
Cholesterol: 35 mg
Sodium: 270 mg
Potassium: 380 mg
Phosphorus: 200 mg
Calcium: 32 mg
Fiber: 2.3 g

325. Slow Cooker Kale and Turkey Meatball Soup

Preparation time: 15 minutes

Cooking time: 4 1/2 hours.
Servings: 4

Ingredients:

- 1/4 cup 1% fat milk
- Whole wheat bread: 2 slices
- 2 cloves of garlic pressed
- 1 cup of ground turkey
- 1/2 of a teaspoon freshly grated nutmeg
- 1 medium shallot finely diced
- 1/4 of a teaspoon red pepper flake
- Kosher salt and freshly ground pepper
- 1 teaspoon of oregano
- 1 egg white
- 2 tablespoons Italian parsley chopped
- 1 tablespoon of olive oil
- 1/2 yellow onion finely diced
- Chicken or vegetable broth: 8 cups
- Kale: 4 cups
- 2 carrots cut into slices
- 1/2 of a cup cheddar grated, extra for garnish

Directions:

1. Take a large mixing bowl, add milk, and let the bread slices soak in the milk.
2. Then, add the garlic, turkey, nutmeg, shallot, red pepper flakes, salt, oregano, pepper, egg, and parsley, and mix carefully with your hands. Help yourself with a scooper to make half-inch balls.
3. After doing this, put a wide skillet on medium flame, heat the olive oil, and then sear the meatballs gently on each side for two minutes. Turn off the heat and set it aside.
4. Add the onion, stock, kale, and carrots to a 5-to-7-quart slow cooker.
5. Add meatballs to the kale, and cook for four hours at low or until the meatballs start floating to the top.
6. Garnish the soup with cheddar grated cheese, red

pepper flakes, and fresh leaves of parsley.

Nutrition Facts Per Serving:

Calories: 457.14 kcal

Total Fat: 23.05 g

Carbs: 40.66 g

Protein: 26.41 g

Sodium: 1200 mg

Potassium: 900 mg

Phosphorus: 160 mg

Conclusion

And there you are at the end of this renal diet book. I hope that both the introduction and, more importantly, the recipes have been to your liking and will be helpful in this new journey of your life.

I want to point out that this book does not replace a doctor's opinion but can help you as a guideline to follow. Your health care provider must advise you on the correct doses of potassium, sodium, and phosphorus to take during the day.

These recipes will surely give you proper support and serve as a starting point to know what to cook and enjoy a meal without giving up anything. In conclusion, I want to wish you good luck and tell you that life is a beautiful gift and we must take care of it...and I am sure you will do it in the best way.

Lightning Source UK Ltd.
Milton Keynes UK
UKHW020653310521
384676UK00011B/712

9 781802 230109